THE
COLOR CODE

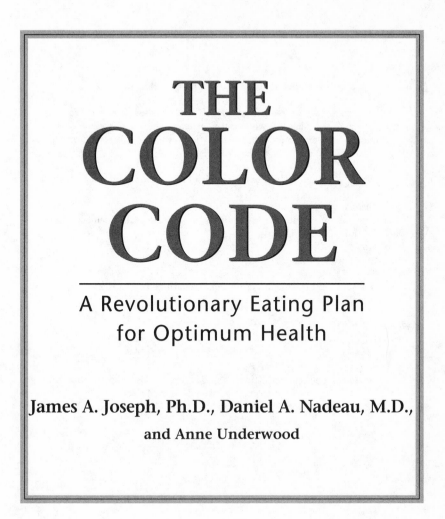

THE
COLOR
CODE

A Revolutionary Eating Plan for Optimum Health

James A. Joseph, Ph.D., Daniel A. Nadeau, M.D.,
and Anne Underwood

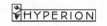 HYPERION

NEW YORK

Produced by The Philip Lief Group, Inc.

Library of Congress Cataloging-in-Publication Data

Joseph, James A.
    The color code: a revolutionary eating plan for optimum health / James A. Joseph,
Daniel Nadeau, & Anne Underwood.
        p. cm.
    Includes bibliographical references.
    ISBN 0-7868-6721-3
        1. Nutrition.   2. Health.   3. Aging—Nutritional aspects.   I. Nadeau, Daniel
II. Underwood, Anne   III. Title.

RA784 .J678 2002
613.2—dc21
                                                                        2001039246

Hyperion books are available for special promotions and premiums.
For details contact Hyperion Special Markets,
77 West 66th Street, 11th floor, New York, New York, 10023,
or call 212-456-0100.

FIRST EDITION

10   9   8   7   6   5   4   3   2

ACKNOWLEDGMENTS

I would like to acknowledge God for His wonderful work in creating the myriad of colorful fruits and vegetables described in this book. I would also like to thank the people in my laboratory—Drs. Barbara Shukitt-Hale, Natalia Denisova, Kuresh Youdim, Antonio Martin, and Donna Bielinski, as well as Mr. Derek Fisher, Ms. Gemma Casadesus, and our outside collaborators Drs. Paula Bickford and Mark Smith—for their great work in elucidating the health benefits of the fruits and vegetables. And I would like to thank my wife, Marlene, for her valuable advice and counsel in my research.   —J. J.

I would like to acknowledge my scholarly mentor and friend, the late Thomas Franklin Grady, Ph.D., the Tenth Viscount Guillamore, whose inspiration remains as constant as the North Star. Special thanks go to Mary E. Fleming, R.D., L.D., who contributed innumerable hours to developing recipes and menu ideas for the program and who helped ensure nutritional balance for each day of the Seven-Day Meal Plan. Thanks also to Bonnie Murray for technical assistance; and to Mary Ellen O'Neill and her colleagues at Hyperion, my heartfelt gratitude for bringing this book to fruition.   —D. N.

There is not enough space here to thank everyone who made this book possible. But I would like to single out a few people for special recognition. First, I would like to thank my ever-loving husband, Ridley Enslow, for his unflagging suppport and his patience during months when he barely saw me. Second, I would like to thank my co-authors, Dan Nadeau and Jim Joseph, for their expert guidance, and Jamie Saxon for her brilliant editing along with Mary Ellen O'Neill at Hyperion for believing in this book and working so hard on it. Third, I must thank the scientists—more than 200 of them—who spent hours on the phone with me, explaining the roles of different phytochemicals, answering questions, and faxing me their research papers. There are too many scientists to name them all, but a few who were of special help were Amy Howell, Willy Kalt, Paul Talalay, Fred Khachik, Jim Duke, Randy Hammond, Jim Demers, Ron Wrolstad, John Folts, Allan Conney, Daniel Nixon, and John Weisburger. Finally, I could never have accomplished this without the cooperation of my editors at *Newsweek* and their willingness to grant me leave to write this book. My profound thanks to them all.   —A. U.

CONTENTS

THINK HEALTH—THINK COLOR!

> "If you don't take care of your body, where are you going to live?"
>
> —Anonymous

LIFE ISN'T A BOWL OF CHERRIES. But maybe it should be. Rich, deep-red cherries, mixed with luscious blueberries and succulent peaches, all bursting with flavor. Or fresh ears of golden corn from a roadside stand, rich with the scents of summer. Or bows and flows of angel-hair pasta, drenched in a tangy red marinara sauce. These foods, so enticing in their colors and scents, are also brimming with the promise of health.

We mean that literally. In the fifth century B.C., Hippocrates, the father of Western medicine, declared, "Let food be your medicine and your medicine be your food." The ancients had keen powers of observation. Pliny the Elder recorded no fewer than 87 medicinal uses for cabbage and 28 for garlic. The Romans found medical applications for lentils, grapes, and raisins.

The sages of old never tested their ideas with scientific studies as doctors do today. But we think they were onto something. Around the world, low-fat diets that are rich in fresh produce contribute to longer, healthier lives. In Japan, where the traditional diet consists of rice, soy, tea, fish, and a rainbow of colorful vegetables, people have the world's longest life expectancy. In rural China, where they eat a similar semi-vegetarian diet, the incidence of heart disease and certain cancers is among the lowest in the world. But a curious thing happens when Asians move to the United States and adopt the standard American diet, with all its high-fat junk food and empty calories. Their rates of cancer and heart disease soar.

The Asians are not alone. The Pima Indians in Arizona did not have a single recorded case of adult-onset diabetes while they sub-sisted on their traditional diet of wheat, squash, beans, cactus buds, squawfish, and jackrabbit. After Uncle Sam started sending surplus meat and cheese, however, their incidence of diabetes began to rise. Later, when they began chowing down on fast foods and typical American junk foods, half the adults over age 35 developed dia-betes. Meanwhile, their Mexican cousins across the border main-tained a traditional diet—and traditionally low disease rates.

How can we explain these medical puzzles? Cutting-edge sci-ence has started piecing the answers together. And though the puz-zle itself is exceedingly complex, the overall picture is pretty plain. It turns out that colorful, fresh produce is a key feature of any diet for optimum health. That's because fruits and vegetables, espe-cially the most colorful ones, contain a bushel of disease-fighting compounds. You don't have to search out Chinese bok choy or the cactus buds of Pima Indians. The Mediterranean diet, with its vibrant palette of foods, offers similar protection. Indeed, almost every colorful food—from fresh-picked apples to cool green kiwis, bright red strawberries, and zesty, ripe oranges—is loaded with disease fighters. Many of them are found in the pigments them-selves. Consider:

- The natural dye that makes tomatoes red may help ward off prostate cancer. A Harvard study found that 10 servings of tomato products a week reduced the risk of aggressive tumors by nearly half.
- The crimson in sour cherries may alleviate your arthritis pain. Researchers in Michigan found sour cherries to be 10 times stronger than aspirin.
- The yellow in corn could protect your eyesight. Repeated studies have found that it helps prevent macular degenera-tion, the leading cause of blindness in people over 65.
- The golden pigment in curry powder can reduce inflamma-tion. Researchers are now studying its potential to prevent colon cancer, which is often linked to inflammation.

- The blue in bilberries, a close relative of blueberries, appears to enhance night vision. During World War II, the Royal Air Force fed bilberry jam to British pilots to aid night missions.
- Perhaps most intriguing of all, the indigo pigments in blueberries may stave off the natural mental decline that occurs as we age. Jim Joseph, one of the co-authors of this book, has conducted groundbreaking research in rats, showing that blueberries slow and even *reverse* some damage to aging brains, improving the animals' short-term memory and coordination.

For these reasons and many more, we're not just speaking metaphorically when we say that these foods are part of a "color code" for healthy living. Many of the ailments that we've come to fear—cancer, heart disease, diabetes, and osteoporosis, among others—are not inevitable at all. They're consequences of how we live and how we eat. By fortifying our diets with colorful fruits and vegetables, we may prevent many of these diseases from striking in the first place. But to do that, we need protective benefits from the full spectrum of brightly hued produce. "It may be that the goal of five fruits and vegetables a day is really about color," says John Sauvé, executive director of the Wild Blueberry Association of North America. "You can paint the image of health, but you need all the colors to do that—red, green, orange, and blue—some of each every day."

Think of it as pigment power.

Food for Life

There are many reasons to eat colorful foods. In addition to pigments, plants contain a broad range of compounds that impart flavors and scents and fight off bugs. Known collectively as *phytochemicals* (from the Greek word *phyton*, "plant"), these chemicals technically include such familiar substances as proteins, carbohydrates, vitamins, and minerals. But in the popular usage—which we will conform to in this book—the word "phytochemicals" usually refers to the other substances that make up the rest of what's in a plant. Plants manufacture those compounds to protect themselves against a variety of dangers, ranging from solar radiation to menacing microbes. The great thing is, these vegetable defenders turn out to protect people, too, against a whole host of ills.

For example, certain phytochemicals activate genes that help the body fight cancer. Scientists are starting to think of them as a form of gene therapy—but before any disease has developed. "Gene therapy has become the buzzword in cancer treatment," says Dr. Andrew Dannenberg, director of cancer prevention at New York Presbyterian Hospital-Cornell Medical Center in New York. "It's high tech and elegant, but it's also expensive and unavailable. On the other hand, each and every day, you eat. It might just be that the most effective form of gene therapy is diet. It can keep you from getting sick in the first place."

With all this health-promoting power, phytochemicals are the most exciting thing happening in nutrition today. For years, we've known about vitamins, minerals, and fiber. Those are all good substances—*great* substances—but now we know there's even more to a healthy diet than vitamins and minerals. There's also the disease-busting strength of phytochemicals. You can't get this protection out of a bottle, but you can get it from a diet rich in colorful produce.

This new way of thinking represents nothing short of a revolution in nutrition. It's not good enough just to extract vitamins and minerals from foods and put them into pills. If you do, you're getting only part of the life-preserving package that nature gave us. You're missing out on a wealth of natural defenders that can help guard against everything from blindness to cancer.

Defensive Eating

It's hard to go wrong if you fortify your diet with colorful foods. Almost every one of them is loaded with disease-proofing compounds. Take blueberries. Until recently, these diminutive fruits were written off as nutritional weaklings. Now scientists are having to eat their words. A USDA database reveals that blueberries contain more than a dozen vitamins and minerals in small amounts. They pack fiber. *And* they contain nearly 100 phytochemicals, including the stubborn dyes that stain your mouth and sometimes your shirt. Just one of these phytochemicals falls into the following protective categories, according to a USDA database: "analgesic, antibacterial, anticancer, anti-inflammatory, antioxidant, antiseptic, antisunburn, antiulcer, [and] immunostimulant." Harness those in your diet, and you've achieved what Elizabeth Ward of the American Dietetic Association calls "defensive eating."

And that's just one fruit. Imagine what you can do with a whole diet full of this brightly colored stuff. People have gotten used to thinking of fruits and vegetables as delivering one nutrient or another. Oranges, vitamin C. Bananas, potassium. But the reality is that every fruit and vegetable is a complex disease-fighting machine. A glass of orange juice contains 170 phytochemicals—not to mention potassium, thiamin, folate, and hefty amounts of vitamin C. Carrots contain a total of 217 compounds. Apples, at least 150. The bottom line is that your mom was right, even if she didn't know why. The old folk wisdom that you should include green and orange vegetables in your daily diet was absolutely correct. It just didn't go far enough. Today we know that you should also include a daily sampling of red, purple, and blue—the more colorful, the better.

Mind-Bending Evidence
With every passing year, mind-bending new evidence adds support to the wisdom of eating a color-packed diet. The truth is that if greengrocers had the marketing muscle of drug companies, we would all be racing to try this miracle regimen. Patients would demand that their doctors prescribe it. Consumers would flock to the produce aisles to snap up these lifesaving foods. We say this with absolute conviction.

We, the three authors of this book, have performed different, but related, work. Jim Joseph has conducted original research on the benefits of the most intensely colored fruits and vegetables. Dan Nadeau has treated patients, using a colorful diet as one path to health. Anne Underwood has combed the published literature on phytochemicals and spoken to hundreds of experts across the country. Again and again, the same bottom line emerges: whole foods—colorful foods—deliver protection against a broad range of ailments. And the reason comes back to the cornucopia of pigments and other phytochemicals they contain.

The research may be complex, but the take-home message isn't. Our philosophy can be summed up in the simplest of mottos: Think health, think color!

The Color Code

This, then, is the heart of the Color Code program—learning to enliven your plate and your palate with these colorful, life-giving foods. For simplicity's sake, we've divided fruits and vegetables into four broad color groups—red, orange-yellow, green, and blue-purple. The goal is to eat foods from each of these groups every day. As nutritionists have known for decades, the greens and oranges contain powerful life-sustaining chemicals, including the carotenoid pigments. The reds and purples have different pigments that are potent antioxidants. And each fruit or vegetable has its own unique complement of phytochemicals—that's what makes a strawberry different from an orange or a grape. Eating from each group helps ensure that you get everything you need. As you read through the "color" chapters, you will quickly start to assemble a mosaic of colorful foods that you don't want to miss.

Of course, fruits and vegetables can't be the only thing you eat. Other foods are essential to a well-rounded diet, too—including whole grains, fish, nuts, and legumes. We discuss all of these in Chapter 6, which presents the Color Code eating program. Many of you will be glad to know that you don't have to become vegetarians to reap benefits. Lean meat—including fish and skinless poultry—can be part of a healthy diet, too. But the more fruits and vegetables you consume, the more disease-fighting phytochemicals you recruit into your own personal defense force. Think of it this way: Each time you pass up a Twinkie or a sugary soda and eat fruit instead, you've just fortified your body with health-giving compounds instead of empty calories. The more colorful your food choices, the better. It's what we like to think of as a fruitful approach that will leave you feeling in the pink, so to speak. But don't take our word for it. Try harnessing some of this pigment power, and see if you don't start feeling fitter.

The best part is that the Color Code eating plan is both fun and delicious. You'll explore new tastes while starting to approach meals in an entirely new way—through maximizing the colors on your plate. As you will see, this also helps you boost your intake of vitamins and minerals. What's to lose? In this book, we will help you get there, with eating tips, a color scoring system, and delicious recipes. So dig in! There's no time like the present to start. As Eubie Blake said on his 100th birthday: "If I'd known I was going to live this long, I'd have taken better care of myself."

NOT BY BREAD ALONE

Eating well is not the only thing you must do if you want to achieve and maintain optimum health. Here are three more:

- Exercise. Physical activity works in many ways to help maintain peak mental and physical performance. Aerobic activity stimulates blood flow, bringing oxygen and nutrients to vital organs, including the brain. Weight-bearing exercise builds bone strength. Stretching improves flexibility and mobility in general. Research shows that exercise can alleviate depression and sharpen mental function. It can also help prevent osteoporosis, diabetes, hypertension, heart disease, and breast and prostate cancers.

  Exercise is so important that the USDA incorporated exercise into its latest *dietary* guidelines. This doesn't mean we all have to become marathon runners. (Lucky for us!) Just 30 minutes of moderate exercise a day will meet the USDA requirement for adults. That half hour can even be broken into three 10-minute segments—and can include housework, climbing stairs, and playing actively with your kids.
- Reduce stress. On a chronic basis, stress can decrease immune function, contribute to atherosclerosis, encourage ulcers, and lead to impotence, among other things. Fortunately, almost any form of stress reduction that you personally find relaxing will help, including exercise, music therapy, yoga, and meditation—even walking the dog. Find something that works for you.
- Avoid smoking. OK, so you already know the dangers of excess alcohol, and you've heard the grim statistics about tobacco—how smoking triples the risk of dying from heart disease and is the single most avoidable cause of cancer (including tumors of

the lung, mouth, throat, esophagus, larynx, pancreas, bladder, and kidney). We hope that anyone who's health conscious enough to be reading this book won't even be tempted to smoke. But just in case, here's some added incentive. Recent research shows that smoking accelerates bone loss, leading to osteoporosis and hip fractures. It impairs circulation, making it more difficult for wounds to heal. And according to scientists, it takes an average of 7 to 10 years off a person's life.

Follow all of these recommendations and you'll be living the full Color Code program—and probably feeling a lot better, too!

Why Plants Are Colorful

To understand why phytochemicals have such powerful effects on the body, it's helpful to know what they do for plants. A good place to start is with pigments. These fall into two main classes, known as *carotenoids* and *anthocyanins*.

The Yellow-Orange Carotenoids

Carotenoids cluster at the yellow-orange-red end of the spectrum. They make corn golden, tomatoes scarlet, and carrots orange. They're also densely packed into leafy greens like spinach, but you can't see them because chlorophyll, with its intense green coloring, masks their hues. In the same way, maple leaves appear green all summer until the autumn cold snaps kill off the chlorophyll, revealing the blazing golds beneath.

Vegetables and autumn leaves aren't the only places we find these pigments. Salmon are salmon-colored because they feed on algae that contain carotenoids. The characteristic hues of lobsters, goldfish, and even flamingos come from the carotenoids in their diets. If a flamingo consumes a low-carotene diet, he grows pale. There are over 600 carotenoids in nature, but only 50 in the human diet—of which 25 or so get into the bloodstream. The most important of these are alpha- and beta-carotene, beta-cryptoxanthin, lycopene, lutein, and zeaxanthin. You'll learn more about each of these in the individual color chapters in this book.

The Red-Blue Anthocyanins

The other major class of pigments are the anthocyanins (from the Greek words *anthos,* "flower," and *kyanos,* "dark blue"). These complete the rainbow spectrum, with hues ranging from crimson and magenta to violet and indigo. These pigments are found throughout the plant kingdom. They make roses red and violets blue—and scientists have honored this association by giving the *anthocyanidins* (the most basic anthocyanins) such floral names as delphinidin, petunidin, peonidin, and rosinidin. Anthocyanins are also widely distributed in the foods we eat. Cherries, plums, red currants, and blueberries all owe their beautiful hues to anthocyanins. There are more than 300 of these pigments, 70 of which have been reported in fruits.

Pigments Are a Plant's Sunblock

These natural dyes aren't there just for decorative purposes, however. They are versatile helpers, serving a vast range of functions. One of the most important of these jobs is to protect plants against damaging sunlight. After all, when the day is a scorcher, plants cannot simply move to a shady spot or apply sunblock. "Plants live in a sea of ultraviolet light that would kill most of us," says Joseph Hotchkiss, professor of food science and toxicology at Cornell University.

For a plant, sunshine is both a blessing and a potential curse. That's because sunlight sustains the life-giving process of photosynthesis. On the other hand, photosynthesis generates enormous amounts of free radicals—those unstable and damaging molecules that you read about in health magazines. Just as free radicals threaten human health, they can damage plants. But carotenoids and anthocyanins are powerful antioxidants that rally to the defense of plants.

Without antioxidant pigments to save them, plants would quickly die. This is not mere theory. Scientists have discovered mutant tomato plants that lack carotenoids in their green leaves. Without these protective pigments, the chlorophyll is rapidly destroyed—and without chlorophyll, the plants themselves cannot live. They wither without forming seeds. They never produce even the tiniest tomatoes.

Flavonoids, Terpenes, and Other Tongue Twisters

As important as they are, carotenoids and anthocyanins are just subgroups in larger classes of phytochemicals. The carotenoids belong to a group of compounds called *terpenes* and *terpenoids*. Anthocyanins come from a group called *flavonoids* (deriving their name from the Latin word *flavus*, "yellow," since some of the first to be identified were yellow). Flavonoids in turn are part of an even larger class known as *polyphenolics*, which are potent antioxidants.

There are also many smaller classes of phytochemicals, including the indoles, saponins, lignans, and tongue twisters like isothiocyanates. These names were obviously devised by scientists, not consumer-friendly focus groups. But the important ones in this book are not all that difficult, so hang on!

Why Do Plants Need These Compounds?

Many of these compounds provide plants with scents or flavors. For example, a carrot tastes sweet because of the natural sugars it contains, but what makes it taste like a carrot rather than a spoonful of the white stuff? Terpenes. The main one in carrots is called terpinolene. Another terpene, called pinene, gives pine needles their characteristic scent. For plants, taste and scent are essential. Colors, fragrances, and tastes help plants attract certain species (such as pollinating bees) and repel others (such as gnawing insects).

Other phytochemicals provide plants with the equivalent of an immune system, fighting off bacteria, viruses, and fungi. Perhaps the best known one is a substance in grapes called resveratrol. It's received a lot of attention in the media for helping to reduce heart disease. But grapes use it to fight off bacterial and fungal infections. Because these microorganisms attack from the outside, most of the resveratrol in grapes is found in the skins—so ignore any nutritional cues from Mae West, who famously told her maid in *I'm No Angel*, "Beulah, peel me a grape." When your mother told you that the skins are the best part of fruit, she was right!

Still other plant-based compounds serve as a form of insect repellent. After all, what self-respecting plant wants to be nibbled to death by insects before it can spread its seed? The organosulfur compounds in onions and garlic are among these pest-control compounds. Some organic farmers even use liquid garlic spray on crops to keep the bugs at bay!

What Phytochemicals Mean to You

Antioxidants in plants function as antioxidants in people. But for the majority of phytochemicals, our bodies have devised different uses from those of plants. For example, the organosulfur compounds in garlic serve as pest-control devices in garlic plants, but in humans they battle heart disease and cancer. "Your basic rule of thumb is this: If a compound has a pungent smell or taste, it's probably biomedically active," says Michael Wargovich, director of basic research at the South Carolina Cancer Center in Columbia, South Carolina.

Strictly speaking, scientists do not consider phytochemicals to be nutrients. Nutrients are things like proteins, fats, and carbohydrates that the body uses to generate energy or build cells. They also include substances like vitamins, with which known deficiency diseases are associated, such as scurvy (a vitamin C deficiency) or rickets (lack of vitamin D). Despite this, the term "phytonutrient" has begun to creep into use along with "phytochemical," as scientists become increasingly aware of the crucial role these compounds play in promoting health. "The human body evolved with most of those chemicals," says botanist James Duke, author of *The Green Pharmacy* and compiler of a massive USDA phytochemical database. "That's why you need them in your diet. Cancer in many cases is a deficiency of antioxidants. So is heart disease. Scientists are starting to think of these diseases as a shortage of phytochemicals."

There are many ways that phytochemicals promote health. But three of the most important ones are antioxidant power, anti-inflammatory strength, and the ability to boost our bodies' natural detoxification systems. We will briefly explore each in turn.

The Disease-Fighting Power of Antioxidants

Just as antioxidants protect plants, they literally save people's lives every day. Oxygen enables us to breathe, think, move, and exist. But as our bodies utilize oxygen, they also turn some of it into free radicals—oxygen molecules that are unstable because they have an unbalanced number of electrons. To stabilize themselves, oxygen radicals need to steal extra electrons, and their targets are generally innocent, law-abiding molecules nearby. In effect, antioxidants are the cellular police force that stops these crimes before they can happen. But antioxidants can only accomplish this task if there are enough agents on the force to outnumber the bad guys, enabling them to move in and "quench" free radicals before they can do harm. We will never get rid of free radicals. They're part of life. But we can reduce the "oxidative stress" they cause if we ingest enough antioxidants.

If you want to see antioxidants at work, one place to look is your own kitchen. If you've ever sliced an apple and watched it turn brown, you've seen the effects of oxidation. But what if you dip the apple slices in lemon juice first, as many recipes recommend? Then you can boldly let the apple slices sit out and dare them to turn brown. The vitamin C in the lemon juice is a potent antioxidant, and it will intercept the oxygen before it can strike the fruit.

In the same way, antioxidants in the body trap free radicals before they can damage our cells. This activity helps prevent a range of diseases. Cancer can result from free-radical attacks on DNA, the genetic blueprint of the entire body. Heart disease may follow from oxidation of "bad" cholesterol, also known as low-density lipoprotein, or LDL. Cataracts can come from repeated attacks on proteins in the lens of the eye. Even sunburn and wrinkled skin are the result of free-radical damage. "The damage to DNA is essentially the same as the damage caused by radiation," says Dr. Denham Harman of the University of Nebraska, the father of the free-radical theory of aging. "It's like being irradiated by an X-ray machine. But we can prevent that by the antioxidants we take in." Many of the strongest antioxidants are the protective pigments in fruits and vegetables.

The Body's Natural Detox Crews

Just as our bodies have their own equivalent of a law-and-order force, they have an elaborate cleanup crew for toxic waste disposal. And guess who many of key players are? Phytochemicals. The saponins in legumes scoop up cholesterol in the intestinal tract before it can be absorbed into the bloodstream. Like efficient little conveyor belts, they keep the cholesterol moving right on through the system and out the other end.

Other members of this cleanup crew sweep away potential carcinogens. Many cancer-causing nitrosamines are formed in the body when nitrogen compounds link up with parts of proteins

called amines. But two of the phytochemicals found in tomatoes—
p-coumaric acid and chlorogenic acid—can intervene to stop the
process. These efficient sweepers whisk away the nitrogen compounds before they can bind with amines. The same protective
compounds are found in many fruits and vegetables, including
strawberries, carrots, pineapples, and green peppers. That's one
more reason to dig into the red, orange, yellow, and green food
groups.

Still other toxic-waste fighters clear away carcinogens that
have already formed. For example, a compound called sulforaphane in broccoli activates the genes that make crucial detoxification enzymes. These enzymes are like the janitors that gather
up garbage and put it out for trash collection. They take an insoluble carcinogen in the cell and hook it up to a soluble compound,
which can then dissolve in the bloodstream. The blood proceeds
to clear it away like a heap of rubbish on trash night.

The Anti-inflammatory Brigade

Inflammation is not necessarily a bad thing. In fact, it's essential to
repairing injuries. When you cut yourself, the body rushes in an
emergency medical team of inflammatory chemicals. This emergency crew calls in an extra supply of nutrient-rich, oxygenated
blood to repair the injury. It also brings in white blood cells to
fight infection and increases fluid levels to cushion the damaged
cells. (That's why the injury looks red and swollen.) Inflammation
is a necessary fact of life.

But when it gets out of hand, look out! Evidence is mounting
that chronic inflammation may contribute to certain types of cancer. The reasons are not fully understood. But inflammation leads
to the release of damaging substances that can encourage cell proliferation in tumors. Inflammation also plays a role in heart disease and stroke. "The bottom line is that atherosclerosis is not just
a disease of cholesterol," says Dr. Paul Ridker, a cardiologist at
Harvard Medical School and director of the Center for Cardiovascular Disease Prevention. "Inflammation turns out to be part and
parcel of the process." Recent studies have suggested that blood
levels of an inflammatory chemical called C-reactive protein can
predict heart-attack risk even better than cholesterol. The two

measurements together are a much more reliable indicator of risk than cholesterol alone.

Inflammation may even play a role in the development of Alzheimer's disease, although the evidence is not as clear. A large study at Duke University is tracking pairs of identical twins to determine why two people with identical genes do not develop the highly hereditary disease at the same time. Among these twins are Doris and Dorothy Wyne, aged 78. Doris has had the disease for eight years. Dorothy doesn't show a sign of it. One possible explanation: the anti-inflammatory drugs that Dorothy takes for her arthritis. "Inflammation is bad news," sums up William A. Pryor, director of the Biodynamics Institute at Louisiana State University in Baton Rouge.

The good news is that substances in food can help fight inflammation. In the lab at least, many phytochemicals seem to be potent anti-inflammatories. One of the strongest is curcumin, the yellow pigment in the curry spice turmeric. In animal tests, it helps prevent tumors. Other natural anti-inflammatories include the carnosol in rosemary and the red anthocyanin pigments in tart cherries.

Can You Get All This Good Stuff From Supplements?

The short answer is no. Scientists don't even know what all the phytochemicals are yet. But even if they did, these compounds appear to function in vast, synergistic networks. Bottling a single chemical defeats the whole purpose. Could Michael Jordan have single-handedly won the NBA playoffs without the rest of the Bulls? The idea is ludicrous. When it comes to phytochemicals, you want the whole team on your side, too, not just an isolated MVP. You want the myriad of antioxidants, the full host of health-preserving chemicals. "To take one out of context and put it in a pill makes little or no sense, when there are thousands of compounds in plants that are associated with lower disease rates," says Cornell University biochemist T. Colin Campbell, who helped conduct the longest-running study to date of the Chinese diet and disease prevention. The only way to take advantage of them all is by eating a diet rich in brightly colored fruits and vegetables, not popping supplements every day. Says Campbell: "There are no magic bullets."

The More Colorful, the Better

One of the most exciting lessons to come out of all this new research is the realization that the greatest number of healthful compounds can be found in the most colorful foods. Perhaps the first inklings of this truth came from Harry Steenbock, a biochemist at the University of Wisconsin way back in 1919. Steenbock fed rats one of two diets—a "white diet," consisting of white corn, potatoes, and parsnips, or a "yellow diet," rich in yellow corn, sweet potatoes, and carrots. "The rats on the yellow diet thrived in their normal, ratlike way," says Philipp Simon, a research geneticist at the University of Wisconsin in Madison. "Those on the white diet died in three months." That's because they lacked the crucial carotenes.

People, too, need to load up their diets with colorful foods. Virtually all fruits and vegetables—pale and vibrant alike—have something to recommend them. But vegetables that are darker not only have more antioxidant pigments—they often have more vitamins as well. For example:

- Butternut squash delivers more carotenes—and hence, more vitamin A—than summer squash, which is essentially white on the inside.
- Pink grapefruit gives you the antioxidants lycopene and beta-carotene, which are missing from white grapefruit.
- Deep green romaine lettuce contains more B vitamins than pale iceberg. "Eat a whole cup of iceberg and you get ten percent of the U.S. Recommended Daily Allowance for . . . well, nothing," says nutritionist Bonnie Liebman of the Center for Science in the Public Interest.
- Even red wine packs a more potent antioxidant punch than white.

Just as Nature Made Them

The best way to eat all of these foods is just as nature made them, in the least processed form available. In short, baked potatoes with the skins are more nutritious than potato chips, which have been peeled, chopped, fried, and salted. Whole apples beat apple juice, which has been peeled, cored, and pressed. Brown rice beats white. Whole strawberries beat jam.

In part, that's because unhealthy fats, sugar, and salt are added in processing. And in part, it's because healthy skins and outer coatings are stripped away. What are you losing with the skins? Among other things, color. Clearly the most colorful part of an apple is the peel. The most vibrant part of a zucchini or even a blueberry is its skin. (Check the inside of a blueberry, and you'll see that it's green, not anthocyanin-rich blue.)

Shop for Color
Any fruit or vegetable you buy should be the one with the best color—the reddest strawberries, the blackest blackberries. Shop for broccoli that is a deep, dark green, not tinged with yellow. Search out vibrant scarlet tomatoes, not pale red or greenish ones. There are two reasons for this.

First, as fruits ripen, the pigments themselves become more dense. Blueberries double and triple their anthocyanin content between the time they first turn blue and the time they reach full maturity. Sour cherries show a twentyfold increase. That means more antioxidants for you.

Second, as fruits and vegetables ripen, they increase their stores of vitamins and minerals. By buying the bright crimson strawberries rather than pale, half green ones, you'll not only get more anthocyanins, you'll get more vitamin C, too.

In the quest for good health, you need to arm yourself with the most richly colored fruits and vegetables. It's the Color Code way.

DID YOU KNOW? EVEN WITH CHOCOLATE,
DARKER IS BETTER

Chocolate has been a popular indulgence for centuries. But lately it's become even more tempting, thanks to the discovery that it contains a class of exceptionally powerful antioxidants—namely, a set of flavonoids called *catechins*. These are the same compounds that give tea its antioxidant strength. But not all chocolates have equal amounts.

Dark chocolate has the most. That's because it has the most so-called chocolate liquor, a thick brown paste made from pure ground cocoa beans. At least 35 percent of dark chocolate—and sometimes as much as 75 percent—consists of this chocolate liquor. Milk chocolate is next, containing a minimum of 10 percent. Hot cocoa has very little, because it's so diluted. White chocolate has none. It only earns the name "chocolate" because it contains cocoa butter, the fat from the cocoa bean. "The more of the original bean you have, the better the chocolate is for you," explains chocolate researcher Joe Vinson, professor of chemistry at the University of Scranton.

But don't go hog-wild. Chocolate is still loaded with fat and sugar. Nutritionists recommend no more than one chocolate bar a week.

Go for It!

Are you ready to start packing color into your diet? The first steps are always the hardest. But the concept of maximizing colors is really very simple. Instead of fretting over grams of protein and fat, start thinking whether the plate you've loaded up at the salad bar contains greens, reds, and oranges. That's not too difficult, is it? Ask yourself how you're getting blues and purples, too. Have you eaten any yellows today? Think cornucopias of succulent fruits, kaleidoscopes of life-giving vegetables. Think the Crayola jumbo box of 64 colors! Once you've gotten the hang of it, a brown burger on a white bun starts to look woefully pale. A heap of white French fries doesn't do much to liven up your plate, even with a dollop of ketchup on the side. Drab foods may provide some protein and carbohydrates, plus a smattering of vitamins and minerals. But your health depends on color.

In this book, we will help you to that goal. But first, we'd like to introduce ourselves, so you know a little bit about us and how we came to write this book.

In the Lab with Jim Joseph

I was born in a small town in West Virginia. As I was growing up, we ate a very healthy diet. As it happened, various members of my family had stomach ailments, so my mother kept everyone on a low-fat regimen with abundant fruits and vegetables. Little did I think that this childhood exposure to good nutrition would one day become a part of my research.

My Ph.D. is in the field of neuroscience, the study of the brain—a field that has not traditionally focused on the effects of diet. But after receiving my degree, I took a job at the Gerontology Research Center in Baltimore. There I worked with people like Nathan Shock, the father of modern gerontology. He and his colleagues began to persuade me that it was possible to forestall the deleterious effects of aging. Over the years, it's become clear to me that the most effective way to do that is to exercise regularly, avoid smoking, and eat right—in particular, to consume richly colored fruits and vegetables.

In 1993, I moved to the Jean Mayer USDA Human Nutrition Research Center on Aging at Tufts University in Boston. All my research there has been in rats, who show many of the same effects of aging as humans and at the same relative age. In rodents' brains, just like people's, one of the first things that happens with advancing age is that neurons don't talk to each other as well. That translates into declines in memory and coordination. That's why old folks in the movies are often portrayed as forgetful and unsteady on their feet. But amazingly, my research has shown that foods such as blueberries that are high in antioxidants may help prevent those declines.

My work with blueberries grew out of a carpooling arrangement with my colleague Ron Prior, who was then chief of the polyphenolics laboratory at Tufts. Ron was really excited about a new line of research he had started. He was working with Guohua (Howard) Cao to devise a test that would measure the antioxidant strength of various foods, and he would tell me about it on our rides to and from work. You should have seen their lab. It looked like a salad bar, with strawberries, spinach, garlic, kale, Brussels sprouts, broccoli—everything your mother told you to eat when you were little. They would grind it up, spin it down in the centrifuge, then toss free radicals at it and see how many they could neutralize. They scored the test in ORAC units (short for "oxygen radical absorbance capacity"). One popular magazine dispensed with the scientific terminology and called ORAC units simply "anti-aging points." That's not a bad way to think of ORAC scores, because the evidence is clear that people with the greatest amounts of antioxidants in their diets show the fewest effects of aging.

That's what we've seen with rats in my lab. For the last several years, my colleagues Barbara Shukitt-Hale, Kuresh Youdim, Natalia Denisova, Mark Smith, Antonio Martin, Derek Fisher, Donna Bielinski, and I have been grinding up foods with high ORAC scores and feeding them to aging rats. These rats were already receiving a very healthful diet—better than most Americans routinely consume. On top of that, we added either spinach, strawberry, or blueberry pellets to their diets for two months—the human equivalent of five years. The results? "Color-fed" rats performed significantly better on a test of short-term memory.

We also devised a series of motor-coordination tests that we called the Rat Olympics. In these tests, we made rats walk miniature planks and balance on slowly spinning rods. Amazingly, blueberries were actually able to reverse motor deficits in these aging animals! Blueberry-fed plank walkers retained their balance for 11 seconds—versus just 6 seconds for those on the standard diet. The results of the "lumberjack test" were even more impressive. On average, the blueberry-fed rats were able to stay on for 9 seconds—more than twice as long as the control group on the standard diet.

Does this guarantee that blueberries will have the same effect in humans? Of course not. But I'm not waiting for the evidence to come in. I'm eating blueberries now. They taste good. And compared to some widely touted "anti-aging remedies" like growth hormone injections, they are considerably safer.

DINING WITH JIM

- Of course, there are lots of frozen blueberries in the lab, but the rats usually hog them. We have discussed this with the rats and they said that since they are the ones running the mazes and doing the motor tasks, they should get the first crack at the blueberries. We scientists do get the leftover berries that remain when we switch varieties, but mostly I have to rely on the market for my fresh fruit.
- I find that eating out for lunch every day is expensive, and you don't always know how the food is prepared, so I keep a supply

of soups in my office at Tufts. I also stash jars of roasted peppers, eggplant, and marinated artichoke hearts on the bookshelves. And I keep walnuts or pistachios around for snacks in order to get my daily share of nuts. (This does not include the ones who are always coming into my office to bother me.)

- For dinner, I like couscous or rice topped with browned soy "meat" and roasted veggies—including red peppers, portobello mushrooms, onions, and garlic. This makes a great topping for pizzas as well. There are always lots of onions and garlic in what I prepare.
- My wife, Marlene, and I also try to eat a couple meals a week with spinach in them. A large baby-spinach salad is one option we like. We also enjoy spinach calzones, spinach lasagna, or a tasty Greek spinach pie with feta cheese and mushrooms.

From the Wilds of Maine: Dan Nadeau

My mother has a strong work ethic. That may be how I ended up where I am today. When I was a teenager in Fort Kent, Maine, way up near the Canadian border, she thought I should work during the summer rather than lazing through the warm, sunny days fishing, hiking, and rock climbing. As it happened, we had a small commercial space attached to our house. No one was using it at the time, and the natural foods movement was catching on, so I decided to set up a health foods store there. It was called Nadeau's Natural Foods and was strictly a low-budget affair. But I was excited about it. Not only did I have my own business at age 17, but I also felt I was providing foods that people in town couldn't ordinarily find. I bought a mill and sacks of grain, so customers could walk out with fresh stone-ground flour. I lined the wooden shelves with heavy glass pickle jars and filled them with brown rice and lentils, black beans, and nuts. I also sold teas and cheese and lots of books. My customers ranged from lawyers' wives to backpackers who were trying to escape civilization in the wilds of northern Maine.

In a small town, business was often slow, but I was never bored. On sunny afternoons, I would sit outside reading the books

I carried in the shop—books like *Diet for a Small Planet* by Frances Moore Lappé and *Sugar Blues* by William Dufty. I was amazed to read that Einstein was drawn to vegetarianism. "Nothing will benefit human health and increase chances for survival of life on Earth as much as the evolution to a vegetarian diet," he said. For me—raised on beef at almost every meal—this came as quite a revelation.

After college, I followed my interest in diet to Tufts University, where I received both a master's degree in nutrition and an M.D. I later returned to Maine and became an endocrinologist in Bangor, working primarily with diabetes patients. In perhaps no other medical discipline is the effect of diet as obvious. Adult-onset diabetes is usually the direct result of overeating and indulging too often in foods laden with saturated fat, sugar, and highly refined grains. Once patients have developed diabetes, Western medicine can manage the symptoms, but it cannot cure the disease. Why not prevent it in the first place by eating right?

The more I look at other conditions, the more it becomes obvious to me that diet can help. We spend tons of money on high-tech medical procedures, but if we paid more attention to food and exercise, many of them wouldn't be necessary. That's certainly true of heart disease. Take bypass surgery—known in the medical jargon as coronary artery bypass graft, or CABG (pronounced "cabbage"). When David Letterman returned to his show after quintuple bypass surgery, he spoke of the importance of keeping the coronary arteries clear. "It's Con Ed," he said, comparing these arteries to the local gas and electric company. "If they don't deliver, it's lights out, my friend." But why let our arteries clog up in the first place? Isn't it easier to eat cabbage first than to undergo CABG later?

I use my knowledge of nutrition every day with virtually every patient. I talk about diet through the ages. Humans evolved to be omnivorous. But throughout most of history, people did not have steady access to large amounts of meat. Out of necessity, every major civilization in the past has had a semi-vegetarian diet. Only in recent times have we had so much wealth that we can kill the fatted calf every day. It's catching up to us now, in the form of diabetes, heart disease, and cancer. But we don't have to be passive victims to these modern plagues. By eating right, we can dramatically reduce our chances of suffering all these diseases and more. The latest research—much of it from Jim Joseph's lab—indicates that diet may even help protect the brain as we age. Jim has made national news with his remarkable discovery that blueberries, with their high antioxidant potential, can actually improve memory and motor control in aging rats.

I'm putting all this to work in my own life. I follow a diet that is heavily based on whole grains, fruits, and vegetables (and when in restaurants, fish). It may sound boring, but it isn't. You just have to learn to make good food palatable. It's like relearning lessons from your childhood—relearning how to cook and eat. I start off the day with a delicious blueberry smoothie for breakfast. So do many of my patients—and all the nurses in my office. You can, too.

DINING WITH DAN

- Breakfast to me means blueberry smoothies—made with wild Maine blueberries, of course, since I live in Maine. You'll find the recipe on page 290, but the essential ingredients are soy milk, frozen blueberries, a banana, and flaxseed. For variety, I'll sometimes throw the banana in the microwave for two to three minutes to give it a slightly caramelized flavor. If it's a cold morning and I need a more hearty breakfast, I'll sometimes pour the smoothie on top of oatmeal. I drink a ton of this stuff.

- I eat kale on a regular basis—especially organic kale, which I find has a better flavor. I'll sauté some garlic in olive or canola oil, then add the kale and a touch of water. Sprinkle with soy sauce, and it tastes awesome.

- I snack on seeded red grapes. I feel like a Roman emperor when I pop grapes into my mouth. I buy red grapes, because they require fewer pesticides to grow. I also try to find seeded grapes, because the seeds are actually good for you.

- I became a huge fan of mango drinks when I backpacked through Pakistan and India after college. I would buy these drinks at little roadside stands. Today I'm appalled that I drank them off the street like that, but when it's 95 degrees outside and you're 21 years old, you take chances. I make my mango drink today with fresh or frozen mango, plus soy milk.

A Reporter's Perspective: Anne Underwood

My first clue about the relationship of diet to health came from my mother, a lifelong vegetarian. Although she grew up in a household where dinner was synonymous with meat, she put her foot down at age four and declared that she was only going to eat vegetables. Her philosophy at that age had no deep moral or religious underpinnings. She just knew she didn't like beef.

It's paid off. My mom doesn't come from a family with longevity in its genes. Her father died of heart disease at age 55. Her grandfather succumbed to a stroke at 64, and her grandmother to cancer in her early 50s. By contrast, Mom is still going strong at age 85. Of course, a single person's experience doesn't prove much in scientific terms. Perhaps her good health is only due to general trends toward longer life. But she's outlived her brother and every one of her childhood friends. What's more, she is in good health and high spirits, with none of the ailments that plague so many others at her age. I believe it's the vegetables.

Since I started writing about health and medicine for *Newsweek,* I've read hundreds of studies showing that people who eat the most fruits and vegetables have a lower incidence of everything from strokes and heart attacks to cancer and diabetes. Just as all roads lead to Rome, all health stories seem to lead right to the same bottom line: proper diet and exercise.

Several years ago, my colleague Geoffrey Cowley and I wrote a cover story about centenarians, or people who live to 100 and beyond. They were folks like Angeline Strandal. At age 104, she was still a feisty character. She refused to go to doctors. "If they start poking around you, they'll only make you sick," she told me. But when you're in her kind of health, who needs doctors? The last time she was seriously ill was 1925, when she had her appendix out. Her key to longevity? Among other things, she said, "I'm a vegetarian, more or less. That's one of my good qualities."

A few years later, I spoke with Dr. Leila Daughtry-Denmark. At 102, she was the oldest practicing physician in the country—and had "no intention of retiring." As far as she was concerned, a vacation meant nine holes of golf, not a rest on the couch. Of course, proper diet was one of the keys to her good health. "If you don't eat right, nothing works right," she told me. As far as she was concerned, meals should include beans and nuts, mounds of leafy greens, pots full of homemade vegetable soup, and fresh herbs from the garden, along with basics such as meat and potatoes. As a prescription for fending off infirmity, it seemed to be working for her. She often put in a 12-hour workday—and would see patients at 2 A.M. in an emergency. "I'd rather be working than watching TV," she said.

I found that I couldn't do this kind of reporting for years without making some significant changes in my diet. There was a time in my early 20s—I hate to admit it—when a friend and I jokingly concocted the chocolate diet. It was based on the obviously false premise that there are two essential food groups—chocolate and not chocolate—and that in order to have a balanced diet, one must have some of each every day. I've come a long way since then.

Today I make frequent trips to my neighborhood greengrocer, Sobsey's Produce in Hoboken, New Jersey. There Michael Sobsey and his brother-in-law Mac Ayoubi stock a mouthwatering array of colorful fruits and vegetables—always the finest available, much of it organic. They are constantly challenging my husband, Ridley, and me to try different foods, from passion fruit to blue potatoes. Recently, they had a shipment of cherimoyas, a South American fruit that is now being grown in California. We'd never heard of cherimoyas before, but Michael told us how to make them into a delicious Southwestern-style salad, with mesclun greens, red and orange peppers, red onions, and julienned strips of free-range chicken. The dressing called for orange juice instead of vinegar and was seasoned with honey and fresh jalapeño peppers. It turned out to be a fabulous blend of flavors—the creamy sweetness of the cherimoya balancing out the onion, the honey softening the sting of the jalapeño. And best of all, this salad created a colorful dinner that covered three color groups at once—red, orange, and green. (I was tempted to throw in some blackberries, just to achieve the goal of four color groups in one dish, but we saved the blackberries for dessert instead.) My husband and I love colorful meals that are a feast for the eyes as well as the palate. I predict you'll be searching out colorful recipes, too, by the end of this book.

DINING WITH ANNE

- I adore soups. I'm not talking about your garden variety canned soups here, but scrumptious veggie purées. One of my favorites is a delicious butternut squash soup with apples, onions, and curry powder. (Hint: Microwave the squash first to soften it up.) Restaurant soups usually have too much cream for my taste. But one cream-free soup you can count on is gazpacho, a tangy blend of tomatoes, onions, peppers, cucumbers, garlic, and oil.

- I like a mid-afternoon snack, so almost every morning before work I wash some blueberries or strawberries and pack them in a plastic container to bring to the office. They're antioxidant champions and taste so good, too. The fresh scent that wafts out of the container when I open it always gives me a small thrill.

- Many years ago, when there was still a Soviet Union, I lived there for six months. It never ceased to amaze me, how grocery stores had such meager selections, and yet people would prepare such delicious meals. The magic ingredient in many cases turned out to be fresh dill. Today I use it whenever I can—on salads, sliced cucumbers, borscht, salmon, potato salad, you name it. In fact, I use fresh herbs in general as much as possible. As far as I'm concerned, fresh basil and dill are two of life's greatest pleasures— and unlike chocolate, they're fat-free.

- I acquired a love of vegetable appetizers on travels through Turkey. What I didn't acquire was time to cook them all when I got home. The exception is hummus. In my version, which I learned from the chefs at *Newsweek,* all you have to do is toss canned chickpeas, minced garlic, and olive oil into the food processor, along with a dash of soy sauce and some white pepper. This version has a nuttier flavor than most commercial hummus, which contains lots of tahini. For an extra zing, throw in . . . fresh dill.

One Final Word

Scientific research is a long, arduous process. A single study does not make scientific truth, even though the media often report it that way. It takes dozens of studies on thousands of people to figure out whether the bulk of the evidence lies in one direction or the other. Many of the studies that we cite in this book are cutting-edge science. By definition, that means that there isn't an enormous body of research to back them up. That also means that scientists may discover over time that this or that compound is not as effective as they first thought. For example, high-ORAC foods are potent antioxidants in the lab, but no one can guarantee yet that they provide the same level of protection throughout the body. "The body isn't like a glass of water that antioxidants dissolve evenly throughout," says Dr. Edward Giovannucci of Harvard Medical School. "Certain antioxidants appear to be very specific in the organs they protect." An antioxidant that works well in the blood may do nothing for the brain or the skin. Scientists are only just now beginning to unravel these mysteries—and until they learn more, it will be hard to make definitive statements about many foods and phytochemicals.

There is, however, one statement that we can make with absolute certainty. A low-fat diet that includes a healthy dose of fruits and vegetables can save lives. That's been shown time and time again.

- A powerful Harvard study found that out of 114,000 doctors and nurses, those who consumed five to six servings of produce a day reduced their risk of stroke by 31 percent, compared with those who ate the least of these foods.
- A study of 800 older Dutch men found that those who consumed the most onions, apples, and tea lowered their risk of fatal heart attacks by 70 percent over those who consumed the least.
- Based on numerous studies, the American Institute for Cancer Research estimates that a diet rich in fruits and vegetables could reduce cancers by 30 to 40 percent.

"What's crystal clear is that populations who exercise regularly and eat low-fat, high-produce diets have multiple health benefits," says Dr. Michael Thun, vice president of the American Cancer Society. "These include reduced risks of heart attack and stroke, diabetes, obesity, and various cancers. It's that simple."

The Color Code presents this message in a fresh and unique way, with its focus on color. But the message itself is not new. If you examine the diet books of Dean Ornish, Andrew Weil, Nathan Pritikin, and Michael Roizen, you will find that they share an emphasis on fruits, vegetables, and whole grains. Even Robert Atkins, the most famous proponent of a low-carbohydrate diet, is now incorporating pigment-rich foods into his program, with the recognition that these foods simply can't be ignored—carbs or no carbs.

Phytochemicals are a large part of the reason why fruits and vegetables demand attention. In this book, we present the latest findings about them not so that you will rush out and buy the latest supplement—or even load up your diet with a single food that's rich in a given compound. We present these findings to paint in glorious detail the full, vibrant picture of healthy foods, with compelling reasons why you need all these colorful foods in your diet.

In this century, we've made major strides in public health. Through sanitation and medical advances, developed countries have practically eliminated the infectious diseases and complications of childbirth that used to kill people at an early age. We've done a great job in extending more lives out to the far end of the expected human life span. But that's only half the battle. Now it's time to work on increasing the *health* span. And one of the best ways to do that is with a colorful diet.

RED

2

OF ALL THE COLORS, red is the premier attention getter. Who can ignore a sleek red dress or heart-stopping red lipstick? Doesn't a red Ferrari turn heads? That flashy, look-at-me quality is the reason why stop signs, alarm boxes, and fire engines all are red.

Red foods should grab your attention, too, because they're exciting. Not only do they add visual appeal to a drab dinner, but they also add a plateful of disease-fighting pigments, including cherry red anthocyanins, beet red betacyanins, and tomato red lycopene. Together with the other nutrients in red foods, these pigments mean protection. Of the top 20 antioxidant fruits and vegetables, seven are red:

- Strawberries
- Cranberries
- Raspberries
- Cherries
- Red grapes
- Beets
- Red peppers

That bevy of red beauties tells you something. Reds are as essential to the daily diet as greens and yellows. As you start adding scarlet and crimson to your palette of colorful foods, here are some top ruby reds to ponder.

STRAWBERRIES

Strawberries at a Glance
- Pigments: anthocyanins (four forms of pelargonidin and one of cyanidin)
- Other phytochemicals: ellagic acid, caffeic acid, ferulic acid, glutathione, lignans
- Serving size: one cup (or 8 medium strawberries)
- Vitamins and minerals per serving: C (140% of the Daily Value), folate (7% DV), potassium (7% DV), iron (4% DV), calcium (2% DV)
- Fiber per serving: 14% DV
- ORAC score: 1,540

Heart-shaped and red, the strawberry is an obvious symbol of love. In the language of medieval symbolism, it represented perfection and righteousness. Strawberries were served at important state occasions to promote peace and prosperity. In France, strawberries were traditionally regarded as an aphrodisiac. So great was the belief in their powers that newlyweds were served delicate red strawberry soup. And if a man and woman split a double strawberry, custom held that they would fall in love.

Not only were strawberries thought to encourage amorous attentions, they were also believed to possess healing properties. In 1597, the English herbalist John Gerard wrote that ripe strawberries "coole heate of the stomack and inflammation of the liver." Some hospitals in Europe cultivated the plant in their herb gardens to ensure a steady supply.

Until recently, scientists might have dismissed all this lore as a lot of hocus-pocus. But now we know that there really is reason to believe in the healing power of strawberries. Sadly, they won't guarantee success in love. But if it's antioxidant protection you're looking for, there are few better foods. In the ORAC test at Tufts, strawberries ranked fourth among fruits, thanks in part to their bright red pigments. Now that's something to love!

The Top Antioxidant Fruits and Vegetables

By including antioxidants in your diet, you can help reduce "oxidative stress," or the damage caused by oxygen radicals. Ronald Prior, who helped devise the ORAC test, recommends consuming at least 3,500 ORAC units a day. That's not hard if you start with a serving or two of strawberries. Here is a list of the top antioxidant foods that Prior and Guohua Cao have tested so far. (Dried fruits and garlic are listed separately because they contain relatively little water and therefore have an unfair advantage when ORACs are considered on an ounce-for-ounce basis.) Note: The ORAC values of individual fruits and vegetables can vary, according to growing conditions.

Dried Fruits		Seasonings	
Prunes	5,770*	Garlic	1,939*
Raisins	2,830		

Fresh Fruits		Vegetables and Legumes	
Blueberries	2,400*	Watercress	2,223*
Blackberries	2,036	Kale	1,770
Cranberries	1,750	Spinach, raw	1,260
Strawberries	1,540	Asparagus	1,241
Raspberries	1,220	Brussels sprouts	980
Plums	949	Alfalfa sprouts	930
Avocado	782	Broccoli florets	890
Oranges	750	Beets	840
Red grapes	739	Red bell peppers	731
Cherries	670	Kidney beans	460

*measured in ORAC units per 100 grams (about 3.5 ounces) of food
Sources: Boxin Ou, Brunswick Labs (watercress and asparagus); Ronald Prior and Guohua Cao, USDA-Agricultural Research Service (all other foods)

Jim Joseph's Antioxidant Defense

In 1997, Jim came up with a groundbreaking idea: He wanted to see whether strawberries, with all their antioxidant activity, could help protect aging brains. It seemed logical that they would. The brain is a hotbed of free-radical activity. All that thinking that goes on upstairs requires energy. But in burning glucose for fuel, our brains also produce free radicals—untold zillions of them over the course of a lifetime. As we age, we seem to become more sensitive to their damaging effects. It's not clear why. Are we generating more free radicals? Or do we have fewer antioxidants to protect ourselves? The jury is still out. But Jim reasoned that if we want to protect our minds as we age, high-ORAC foods might help. As he saw it, loading up on antioxidant foods was, well, a no-brainer.

Jim joined forces with Paula Bickford at the University of Colorado Health Sciences Center to put the theory to the test. They first placed rats in chambers containing pure oxygen. Pure oxygen may sound like a good thing, but it isn't. Doctors used to put premature babies in oxygen tents. The result was often blindness. Adults in intensive care who breathe pure oxygen through ventilators can develop a problem called acute respiratory distress syndrome. The lining of their lungs becomes damaged, the air sacs fill with fluid, and the patients have extreme difficulty breathing. "The fact is that we evolved to live in an atmosphere of about 20 percent oxygen," says Bickford. "One hundred percent oxygen is toxic. It generates an excess of free radicals."

She and Jim hypothesized that putting rats in special chambers with 100 percent oxygen for 48 hours would mimic the effects of aging in the brain. And that's exactly what happened. After 48 hours, the scientists removed the rats and monitored the level of activity in their brains. It had decreased substantially. The rats seemed to have aged from 6 months to 18 months overnight, judging by their performance on certain brain tests. In human terms, they'd gone from the equivalent of 18 years old to 60 in those brain functions. (Thankfully, the damage reversed itself after a day or two in normal air again.)

What Happens When You "Color-Feed" the Brain?

Now here's the interesting part. The researchers performed the same experiment with a second group of rats, but fed them for two months on strawberry-fortified diets before exposing them to the pure oxygen. When these "color-fed" rats came out of the oxygen chamber, their brains looked normal. They showed no decreased activity at all. None! The same thing happened with rats fed on blueberries and spinach. All three foods were extremely effective in preventing oxidative damage.

Does this mean that strawberries, spinach, and blueberries will protect human brains against aging? Unfortunately, we don't know yet, and we can't expose people to pure oxygen to find out. But it seems logical. We know that our bodies can absorb antioxidants from these foods. Ronald Prior and Guohua Cao ran a small test at Tufts on eight elderly women and discovered that special drinks made from strawberry extracts boosted antioxidants in the women's blood by 20 percent. The vitamin C in the strawberries could not be solely responsible. "Vitamin C generally accounts for less than fifteen percent of the antioxidant activity of fruits and vegetables," says Prior. That means that the rest of the antioxidant activity in fresh foods must be coming from phytochemicals, including the anthocyanins that give strawberries their bright red hue.

Be Patriotic: Eat Red, White, and Blue

It shouldn't require a holiday for us to eat right. Still, the American Institute for Cancer Research is hoping that the Fourth of July will encourage people every year to think of red, white, and blue—foods, that is. To get in the mood, nutritionist Melanie Polk at the AICR suggests a festive "flag cake," using blueberries and strawberries to make a health-packed Stars and Stripes. (Hint: Use blueberries to create the field for the "stars." To form the stripes, cut the strawberries in half lengthwise, and arrange them end to end in rows.) Polk makes the recipe even more nutritious by enriching the cake batter with mashed bananas.

"Holidays don't have to mean sinful indulgences followed by crash diets," she says. Not if you maximize your colors, anyway. And don't forget—July is National Blueberry Month.

Strawberry Fields Forever

Pigments are not the only reason to love strawberries. Another compelling reason is the phenolic acids. Just one of them, *ellagic acid*, has been shown to prevent esophageal and colon tumors in animals. According to biologist Gary Stoner, chair of environmental health sciences at the School of Public Health at Ohio

State University, it does this by regulating the levels of two crucial sets of enzymes. The first of these—the so-called *phase 1 enzymes*—help cells convert foods into forms the body can use. Unfortunately, in the process, these enzymes also take a certain number of harmless substances and transform them into carcinogens. But not to worry. That's where the *phase 2 enzymes* come in. They attach the toxin to a soluble compound in the cell, then dump it into the blood to be cleared away like trash on collection night. As long as there's more phase 2 activity than phase 1, your body is protected. The remarkable thing about ellagic acid is that it does both. It handcuffs problematic phase 1 enzymes and boosts detoxifying phase 2's. "It's like a one-two punch," says Stoner. And ellagic acid is the heavyweight that delivers the knockout blow.

In addition to regulating these enzymes, ellagic acid plays another very important role. It encourages *apoptosis*. That's a fancy word for cell death. Cells are programmed to die at a certain age or to self-destruct if they develop abnormally. But cancer cells somehow escape these restraints and just keep on multiplying, like an Energizer Bunny out of control. Ellagic acid, in effect, takes the battery out of cancer cells. "It makes cancer cells learn how to die like normal cells," says Dr. Daniel Nixon, a medical oncologist and president of the American Health Foundation in Valhalla, New York.

Ellagic acid does not work alone, however. Because pure ellagic acid is not well absorbed from the digestive tract into the bloodstream, Stoner began working instead with freeze-dried strawberries and raspberries. In the process, he discovered something interesting: Although there was much less ellagic acid in the freeze-dried berries than in the purified extract, it didn't seem to matter. The berries showed equal or better cancer-fighting prowess, at least when tested in animals. That means that it's not only ellagic acid in strawberries that's protective. Says Stoner, "It's probably a combination of ellagic acid with anthocyanins, ferulic acid, caffeic acid, vitamin C, and other compounds."

Stoner is taking this line of research one step further and beginning preliminary trials in humans. The goal is to give berries to patients with abnormal groups of cells called "premalignant lesions" in the esophagus and colon—then see if the berries help prevent the abnormal cells from turning cancerous. "There is no effective treatment for these lesions at the moment," says Stoner. "All doctors can do is follow the patients clinically and remove the lesions if they progress toward cancer." Dr. Nixon, at the American Health Foundation, is planning similar tests for premalignant lesions of the mouth and cervix. "Are we looking at berries for treatment of cancer?" he says. "Absolutely not. But they could prove useful for prevention."

The True Costs

Dan Nadeau frequently hears this objection when he tells people to eat fresh produce: "But isn't that awfully expensive?" That depends a great deal on how you look at it. Replace a steak dinner with a vegetable curry, and you're bound to come out ahead. Purchase apples rather than processed snack foods, and you'll save—in part because you don't get stuck paying for fancy packaging and advertising. Even pricey fruits are actually a terrific buy, if you consider all the vitamins, minerals, fiber, and phytonutrients you get for your money. Many people spend much more than that on supplements every month. But you literally couldn't purchase all of a strawberry's phytonutrients in pill form, for any price. If you look at it that way, even out-of-season strawberries and raspberries are an incredible bargain!

RASPBERRIES

Raspberries belong to the rose family. That explains why they grow on bramble bushes with prickly stems. But despite these prickles, there are few pleasures on a midsummer's afternoon that are as sweet or as healthful as eating raspberries picked fresh off the bush. Raspberries are one of the top antioxidant foods. They contain the same cancer-fighting ellagic acid as strawberries—except they have 50 percent more of it. They also have double the fiber of strawberries—in fact, more than most other fruits. That's because each raspberry is actually a small cluster of 75 to 125 fiber-rich seeds, with every seed encased in a tiny, juicy lobe of its own. Raspberries also boast hefty portions of vitamin C and folate. Here's a quick profile:

- Pigments: anthocyanins (four forms of cyanidin and two of pelargonidin)
- Other phytochemicals: ellagic acid, caffeic acid, quercetin, kaempferol, benzoic acid, cinnamic acid, ferulic acid, farnesol, geraniol, salicylic acid
- Serving size: one cup
- Vitamins and minerals per serving: C (52% of the Daily Value), A (3% DV), folate (8% DV), potassium (5% DV), iron (4% DV), calcium (4% DV)
- Fiber per serving: 34% DV
- ORAC score: 1,220

That's an impressive list. The only problem with raspberries is that they are fragile and spoil quickly. Like the roses they are related to, they require delicate handling. For best storage, experts advise arranging raspberries unwashed in a shallow pan lined with paper towels and placing them in the refrigerator. Do not wash the berries until just before eating.

If you grow to love them enough, then maybe the next time Valentine's Day arrives, you'll try a quirky gift idea. Instead of chocolates and long-stemmed red roses, send your sweetheart a more healthful gift—red raspberries.

SOUR CHERRIES

Sour Cherries at a Glance
- Pigments: anthocyanins (various forms of cyanidin)
- Other phytochemicals: quercetin, kaempferol, chlorogenic acid, p-coumaric acid, gallic acid, perillyl alcohol, D-glucaric acid
- Serving size: 10 cherries
- Vitamins and minerals per serving: A (17% of the Daily Value), C (12% DV), potassium (3% DV), calcium (2% DV), iron (2% DV)
- Fiber: 4% DV
- ORAC score: 670 (for sweet cherries; not available for sour cherries)

When Bernie Tennes began selling tart red cherry juice at his farmers' market, the Country Mill, in Charlotte, Michigan, he had no idea that it would one day become a top-selling arthritis remedy at his shop. At that time, he mainly ordered it to add flavor to the fruit leathers that he made and sold. It worked fine for livening up the leathers. And when he had extra, he would put it out for sale. But cherry juice wasn't exactly in great demand.

Then one day an elderly woman approached the cash register with two gallons of the stuff. Cashier Marlene Smith couldn't resist commenting on this unusual purchase. "Are you making jelly for a bazaar?" Smith asked, intrigued. The woman chuckled. "Oh my, no, honey," she answered. "I take it for my arthritis. Eight ounces a day." She showed Smith how a year of drinking rich red cherry juice had enabled her to close her gnarled fingers into a fist, a task that had eluded her 12 months before.

That was all Smith needed to hear. She began taking cherry juice for her arthritic hip. "I was taking eight hundred milligrams of prescription Motrin at the time," Smith says. "I was only supposed to be taking three hundred or four hundred. That's how bad I hurt." The megadoses of painkillers were also irritating her stomach. But cherries sounded harmless enough. Smith began her cherry-juice regimen—four ounces in the morning and four at night. Three weeks later, she suddenly realized she hadn't taken any pain pills in the previous two days. "I became a confirmed cherry juice drinker," she says. So did Tennes, who still drinks it "religiously" for his own arthritis.

Word spread quickly, and before long, hundreds of seniors were flocking from the surrounding area for their cherry-juice fix— and even mail ordering it from around the country. Among them:

- The retired dean of the Columbia University School of Public Health bought some for his wife, who had severe osteoarthritis in both knees. "I'm an old skeptic," says Dr. Robert Weiss of Orono, Maine. "But in two days, she was without pain. Her orthopedist had been talking about a double knee replacement, but for now that's not in the cards."
- Jane Saims of Portage, Indiana, used to go to bed every night crying from her arthritis pain. Then she found cherry

juice. Within three weeks, she was up and about, doing all her own housework, tending the garden, and even kneeling again in church. She's so enthusiastic that she started buying the juice in bulk and peddling it to friends. "My new motto is, 'I haven't got time for the pain,'" she says.

- Iris Briski of Machesney Park, Illinois, eats sour cherries rather than drinking the juice. She started with 20 a day to help her gout, but after a year was able to cut down to just 10 cherries every other day—chopped up in her cottage cheese. "I'm thrilled with it," she says. "My husband and kids tell me it's just a placebo, but the pain no longer wakes me up at night. I don't think a placebo could do that."

Does this sound too good to be true? Before we go any further, we must emphasize that this is a folk remedy, not a medically tested treatment. The Arthritis Foundation says there are no clinical trials to support the cherry-juice remedy, only anecdotal evidence. Even Dr. Weiss, the physician whose wife experienced such good results, emphasizes that it's not a cure—just a darn good way to get relief from symptoms. "It won't stop the underlying degenerative process," he says. "The cartilage that cushions the joints will continue to wear down."

Nevertheless, for simple relief of arthritis pain, cherries probably deliver more than a placebo effect. And the reason starts with the pigments that make sour cherries a deep, rich red—specifically, three anthocyanin pigments that have demonstrated potent anti-inflammatory effects. Muraleedharan Nair, professor of natural products chemistry at Michigan State University, put these anthocyanins into a test tube along with enzymes that cause inflammation and watched to see if the pigments would block the action of the enzymes. They did. He tried the same thing with pain relievers like aspirin and ibuprofen. Sweet cherries may work just as well. Although no folk remedy backs their use for arthritis, Nair's latest lab tests show that they have even more potent anti-inflammatory effects.

Cherries May Protect Hearts, Too

Anecdotal reports also claim that cherries—both tart and sweet—can help fight heart disease. Do they? A survey conducted by Wirthlin Worldwide for the Cherry Marketing Institute canvassed 366 cherry growers—people who naturally eat a lot of cherries—and found that they had lower levels of heart disease than the national average. No one has done the rigorous studies to support that claim. But there are at least two possible reasons why cherries might help.

First, they contain strong antioxidants in the form of pigments and other flavonoids, including one especially potent flavone that Nair identified in tart cherries. These antioxidants could help prevent heart disease by blocking the oxidation of LDL cholesterol. That's important, because "bad" cholesterol isn't really bad until it's oxidized. Then it can set off a chain of events that leads ultimately to heart disease.

The second reason cherries may help is the anti-inflammatory power of the anthocyanins. Not only does inflammation contribute to the buildup of plaques, but it also determines the vulnerability of those plaques to rupture. When plaques break open, clots form, leading to heart attacks—and a desperate 911 call.

Sweet Medicine

Cherries may even prove to help fight cancer. Both sweet and tart cherries have been found to contain small amounts of a terpenoid called *perillyl alcohol,* which appears to combat tumors, at least in animals. "If you're a rat with breast cancer, you get better results from perillyl alcohol than tamoxifen," says Michael Gould, professor of oncology at the University of Wisconsin Medical School in Madison. Because perillyl alcohol slows the division of cancer cells and also encourages them to self-destruct, it fights tumor growth in two ways. The results are so promising that Gould has begun very early clinical trials with pure perillyl alcohol in humans. In this preliminary phase of testing, the goal is simply to establish safe dosing levels, but the handful of patients in this trial have shown interesting responses. "One case of advanced colon cancer completely regressed and stayed that way for two years," says Gould. "Several others stabilized. But you have to be careful how you interpret these results, because there are so few cases."

Of course, cherries don't contain enough perillyl alcohol to deliver similar results. But the amount they do supply may be a useful contribution to an all-round cancer-fighting diet—a regimen that's low in fat and high in colorful fruits and vegetables.

TOMATOES

Tomatoes at a Glance
- Pigments: lycopene, beta-carotene, zeta-carotene
- Other phytochemicals: kaempferol, quercetin, *p*-coumaric acid, chlorogenic acid, phytoene, phytofluene, D-glucaric acid, alpha-lipoic acid
- Serving size: one medium tomato
- Vitamins and minerals per serving: A (15% of the Daily Value), C (40% DV), potassium (10% DV), iron (3% DV)
- Fiber per serving: 6% DV
- ORAC score: 189

Few foods have enjoyed such a dramatic change in reputation as the tomato. The plant was cultivated by the Aztecs and Incas as early as A.D. 700. When Spanish missionaries and conquistadors arrived on the scene in the 1500s, they were enchanted with the new fruit and brought *tomatl* seeds back to Europe. Spaniards quickly incorporated tomatoes into their cooking. But outside of Spain and Italy, Europeans were generally more cautious. That's because the reigning nutritional theory of the day held that the diet should contain a balance of "hot" and "cold" elements—and tomatoes were deemed dangerously, even lethally, cold. People grew tomatoes in countries like England, but mainly for their decorative value.

By the late 1700s, tomato-phobia was waning. Still, it took a daring fellow by the name of Colonel Robert Gibbon Johnson, president of the Salem County Horticultural Society in New Jersey, finally to end the suspicion surrounding tomatoes. In 1820, Johnson staged a public demonstration on the steps of the Salem

County courthouse in which he ate not one, but an entire basket of tomatoes. Some 2,000 spectators arrived to watch him commit suicide with this foolhardy act. To everyone's shock, he lived. So did the tomato in American cuisine.

The tomato has become one of America's favorite foods. It is also starting to look like a power-packed source of disease protection—and a major reason is the scarlet pigment that gives the tomato its blush.

You Gotta Love Lycopene

That special pigment is *lycopene,* a member of the carotenoid family. Unlike its better-known cousin beta-carotene, lycopene does not convert to vitamin A in the body. This is not a bad thing, however. It means that even more lycopene is available to act as an antioxidant—and lycopene appears to be a potent one. "Lycopene is one of the most potent free-radical scavengers in nature," says Paul Lachance, professor of food science and nutrition at Rutgers University. There's something else interesting about this red pigment. It tends to collect in certain organs of the body, including the lungs and prostate. Not coincidentally, scientists have observed that lycopene consumption seems to reduce levels of cancers in these parts of the body.

Lycopene and Prostate Cancer

Prostate cancer is the most common cancer in American men, with 180,000 new cases diagnosed every year. It's also the second leading cause of cancer deaths for men, claiming 32,000 lives annually. But a tomato-rich diet seems to help. In a 1995 study, Dr. Edward Giovannucci of Harvard Medical School surveyed 48,000 male health professionals to gauge their consumption of 46 fruits and vegetables. He found that men who ate ten or more servings a week of tomato products—raw tomatoes, tomato sauce, tomato juice, and pizza—reduced their risk of prostate cancer by 35 percent. Even more impressive, they reduced their chances of aggressive prostate tumors by nearly 50 percent.

Giovannucci continued to monitor the health professionals and another large group of doctors in the years that followed and refined his results still further. In a 1999 study, he showed that tomato sauce was by far the strongest predictor of low cancer risk, with raw tomatoes placing a poor second. Tomato sauce was so potent, he found, that just two servings a week were enough to reduce the risk. How can this be?

As it turns out, the body is not always able to extract lycopene from raw tomatoes. That's because the pigment is tightly bound up in cell walls and fibers. If digestive juices can't pry it free, then the body can't use it. But boiling the tomatoes down to sauce breaks the cell walls and frees the lycopene. In one German study, researchers fed volunteers 23 milligrams of lycopene a day in the form of either raw tomatoes or tomato paste, which of course is cooked. The researchers then tested the patients' blood and found that lycopene levels were 2.5 times higher in the tomato-paste recipients than in the raw-tomato group.

There's another reason why tomato sauce delivers more lycopene than raw tomatoes: It's prepared with a bit of oil. That's important, because lycopene is not water soluble, but fat soluble. If there isn't a little oil around to transport it, it can't get into the bloodstream. For pizza- and pasta-loving Americans, this is welcome news all around.

Could Ronald Reagan have been on the right track, after all, when he claimed that ketchup is a vegetable?

Tomatoes: Fruit or Vegetable?

Tomatoes are botanically classified as fruit—that is, the seed-bearing part of a flowering plant. In the same way, peppers and avocados are technically fruits, too. But botanical evidence notwithstanding, the United States Supreme Court in 1893 declared that tomatoes were vegetables. In that year, the court heard a case hinging on the question of whether farmers should pay fruit or vegetable freight rates when they shipped tomatoes. Because the tomato is prepared and eaten as a vegetable, the pro-vegetable argument carried the day.

Tomatoes Aren't Just for Men

Any way you slice it, it's not just men who should be eating tomato products. Everyone can benefit. In 1999, Giovannucci analyzed 72 lycopene studies from around the world. In 35 of them, tomatoes significantly lowered the risks of various cancers. (Another 22 studies showed a positive but weak effect.) The best evidence was for prostate, lung, and stomach cancers. But there were also indications that tomatoes could lower pancreatic, colorectal, esophageal, oral, breast, and cervical tumors.

That's an impressive list, but it gets even better. Lycopene appears to protect both hearts and lungs against oxidative damage. In one study, Venket Rao of the University of Toronto found that one to two servings of tomato juice or spaghetti sauce every day for a week decreased damage to proteins, DNA, and cholesterol in the blood of 19 volunteers. A series of European studies suggests that this protection translates into a lower incidence of heart attacks. Similarly, lycopene's antioxidant strength may boost lung power. Lungs are particularly vulnerable to oxidative stress, given their high oxygen exposure. But in a new study, Lenore Arab of the University of North Carolina, Chapel Hill, found that a daily can of V8, along with vitamins C and E, reduced pulmonary functional loss and DNA damage in volunteers who were exposed to elevated ozone levels, which Arab compares to "Mexico City on a bad day." In today's polluted world, why not take advantage of the protection that colorful fruits and vegetables can offer?

Lycopene may even help combat infirmity in old age. The research is still preliminary, but in the now-famous Nun Study, Dr. David Snowdon of the Sanders-Brown Center on Aging at the University of Kentucky assessed 88 Roman Catholic nuns aged 77 to 98 and found that those sisters with the highest blood levels of lycopene functioned the best. They required fewer canes and walkers. They had the least trouble buttoning their sweaters, putting on gloves, and lacing shoes. They were best able to bathe themselves, eat without assistance, and get up out of chairs. Overall, the nuns with the highest blood-lycopene levels were 3.6 times more able to fend for themselves than those with the lowest levels. Snowdon found no such relationship for other antioxidants—namely, vitamin E and beta-carotene—and concluded that lycopene may be "unique" in this regard. More studies are needed to confirm this finding.

Eyes on the Future

Frederick Khachik, a senior research scientist and organic chemist at the University of Maryland in College Park, thinks lycopene may even help vision. At this point, his conjecture is little more than an educated guess. But in a new study, he and his colleagues for the first time identified high concentrations of lycopene in several key parts of the eye. One of these, known as the ciliary body, produces aqueous humor, the clear fluid that fills the eyeball and maintains pressure. The ciliary body also contains the muscles that change the shape of the lens every time it refocuses—say, from the newspaper in front of you to the clock on the wall. Lycopene, with its super antioxidant capacity, could aid both functions by protecting crucial enzymes from oxidation—enzymes that help the ciliary body carry out its tasks. If this is so, then Khachik speculates that lycopene could help forestall or lessen two problems—glaucoma, in which too much pressure builds up inside the eye and can lead to blindness, and presbyopia, which eventually strikes every aging eye, making it hard to focus on small print nearby. So keep that lycopene coming. This is one instance, unlike flash photography, where you don't want "red-eye reduction."

Russian Novels and the "Three Amigos"

As wonderful as lycopene is, it is just one of hundreds of phyto-chemicals in tomatoes. Dr. Steven Clinton, associate director of the Comprehensive Cancer Center at Ohio State University, compares the list to the cast of characters in "a very long Russian novel." "Lycopene may be among the leading characters, but they all play a role," he says. Unfortunately, we are at the beginning of the novel. "We don't know how it turns out," he says. But there is one thing we do know. Just as a Russian novel with only one character would disappoint readers, a tomato with only lycopene in it would not deliver the same health benefits.

So who are the supporting characters in this tomato/novel? In addition to lycopene, tomatoes contain a dozen other carotenoids, including three that have recently intrigued scientists—pale yellow *zeta-carotene* and colorless *phytoene* and *phytofluene*. Exactly what this trio does is not clear, but lab tests show that they're all antioxidants. "We call these carotenoids the three amigos," says Frederick Khachik at the University of Maryland. "They tend to appear together in fruits and vegetables, and all are absorbed at relatively high concentrations. It is a reasonable assumption that they contribute to the biological activity of carotenoids. Exactly how they do that, we don't know yet."

Clinton also thinks the flavonoids play a role. In one new study, he fed rats with prostate tumors either lycopene beadlets or freeze-dried tomato powder. The tomato powder, with its full complement of phytonutrients, outperformed the lycopene, improving survival in the rats by 39 percent on average—versus 17 percent for the pure lycopene. The bottom line is obvious: If you think of the tomato as a novel, you want to read the whole book, not just buy the Cliff's Notes (or lycopene supplements). If you take the shortcut, you'll miss out on a lot of good stuff.

Other Sources of Lycopene

Lycopene is found in relatively few foods. More than 80 percent of lycopene in the American diet comes from tomatoes and tomato products. The rest comes from a handful of other red foods—notably watermelon, pink grapefruit, guava, and papaya. They supply less lycopene in the average American diet, simply because we eat so much less of these fruits than we do of tomatoes. But they are still great ways to boost your lycopene intake—and get other nutrients, too. For example, ounce for ounce, guava contains more vitamin C than any other food in the diet—four times more than oranges!

Red Versus Yellow Tomatoes

There are more than 4,000 varieties of tomatoes. The original ones that were brought to Europe may have been yellow, judging by the Italian name for tomato, *pomodoro* (literally, "golden apple"). But anyone who wants to max out on lycopene will skip yellow tomatoes. They are obviously short on the red pigment.

Otherwise, the red and yellow varieties are a tradeoff. Red

tomatoes contain three times more vitamin C and more vitamin B_6, but the yellow ones deliver more niacin and folate. Both contain equal amounts of the orange pigment beta-carotene.

Eat Tomatoes—Say No to Nitrosamines

Other protective phytochemicals in tomatoes include the so-called phenolic acids—specifically, *p-coumaric acid* and *chlorogenic acid*. Like lycopene, they are also antioxidants. But their most important cancer-fighting effect comes from their ability to inhibit the formation of nitrosamines in the body.

Nitrosamines are a powerful group of more than 400 carcinogens. We eat some of them when we buy processed meats in stores. But many more are made in the body itself, when nitrogen compounds, such as nitric oxide, combine with components of proteins called amines. The body makes nitric oxide for a variety of good reasons, including fighting infections. Unfortunately, the excess nitric oxide can then be diverted to form nitrosamines. "That's one reason that infection and cancer often go hand in hand," says Joseph Hotchkiss, professor of food science at Cornell University.

Nitric oxide is also produced by burning tobacco when we smoke cigarettes. By hooking up with nicotine, it then forms one of the most wicked nitrosamines of all—nitrosonicotine, the main carcinogen in tobacco smoke. These carcinogens are nothing to fool around with. Each year, 164,000 men and women are diagnosed with lung cancer. Each year, 157,000 people die from it.

The best way to prevent lung cancer, of course, is to stop smoking—now! But scientists suspect that tomatoes may also aid in prevention, thanks in part to their phenolic acids. As Sharon Begley wrote in *Newsweek:* "The tomato acids act like Dustin Hoffman in 'The Graduate': they grab hold of the [nitric oxide] and whisk it out of the church—er, cell—before it can go through with its chemical marriage to amines." In a small study of 16 men, Hotchkiss found tomatoes to be the second most potent inhibitor of nitrosamine formation in the body, after green peppers. Although they ranked number two, tomatoes are the top nitrosamine-fighting food in the American diet because we eat so many of them. Other good sources of these phenolic acids are pineapples, strawberries, and carrots— "so eat a variety of fruits and vegetables," Hotchkiss advises.

> **Ketchup Trivia**
> The original *ke-tsiap* from Malaysia consisted of pickled shell-fish, not tomatoes. And European and American versions in the 1600s and 1700s were made from pickled oysters or mushrooms. The first recipe for "tomato catsup" did not appear until Mary Randolph's 1824 cookbook *The Virginia Housewife*. But since then it's taken firm hold. Manufacturers today sell about 550 million pounds of ketchup a year—or two pounds for every man, woman, and child in the United States. With all its salt and corn syrup, ketchup may not exactly be health food, but at least it contains lycopene—ounce for ounce, almost as much as tomato sauce.

RED BELL PEPPERS

Joseph Hotchkiss at Cornell found that green peppers were even better than tomatoes at blocking the formation of the wicked carcinogens known as nitrosamines. You can get the same protection from red bell peppers—plus plenty of other good stuff, too. Red peppers have more vitamin C than oranges. They're one of the top ten foods in beta-carotene content—plus they're one of the best sources of the carotenoids lutein, zeaxanthin, and beta-cryptoxanthin. They're also in the antioxidant top ten. This is one health-promoting food you definitely want on your team. Take a look:

- Pigments: lutein, alpha-carotene, beta-carotene
- Other phytochemicals: *p*-coumaric acid, chlorogenic acid
- Serving size: 1 medium pepper
- Vitamins per serving: A (57% of the Daily Value), C (160% DV), folate (3% DV), potassium (3% DV)
- Fiber per serving: 4% DV
- ORAC score: 731

Red peppers, by the way, contain twice as much vitamin C as green peppers, and nine times more vitamin A.

Fortunately, red peppers are versatile enough to be eaten in many different ways. If you eat them raw, they're crisp and sweet. They are also delicious baked and stuffed. But for our money, one of life's most sublime pleasures is red peppers when they're roasted. Nothing perks up an antipasto plate as much. For that matter, roasted red peppers are a terrific addition to braised kale and garlic. Next time you have a summer barbecue, throw some on the grill for a real taste treat.

Here's the simplest way to roast them: Cut off the top (stem side) of the pepper and scoop out the seeds with a spoon. Then slice the pepper lengthwise into strips. Place the strips on the barbecue grill over an open flame. For an additional zing, brush them with a marinade of olive oil, soy sauce, fresh ginger, and garlic. Turn them several times to cook thoroughly on both sides. Before serving, strip off the charred skin. It will peel off easily. (Peppers can also be broiled in the oven—15 minutes on each side. Remove them and cover with towels for 15 minutes before removing charred skins.)

CRANBERRIES

Cranberries at a Glance
- Pigments: anthocyanins (various forms of peonidin and cyanidin)
- Phytochemicals: condensed tannins (also known as proanthocyanidins), quercetin, kaempferol, myricetin, catechin, epigallocatechin gallate, ellagic acid, chlorogenic acid, benzoic acid, lignans
- Serving size: one cup
- Vitamins and minerals per serving: C (22% of the Daily Value), thiamin (2% DV), potassium (2% DV)
- Fiber per serving: 16% DV
- ORAC score: 1,750

Long before European settlers arrived in America, Native Americans were making a food called pemmican. An early form of jerky, it consisted of thin strips of venison pounded with cranberries and fat, then shaped into cakes and dried in the sun. These cakes did not spoil easily and provided convenient sustenance for long trips and cold winters. Even Arctic explorers came to realize their value. Robert E. Peary wrote in his book *The North Pole*, "Pemmican is the most concentrated and satisfying of all meat foods and is absolutely indispensable in protracted arctic sledge journeys." The reason pemmican kept so well was the cranberries. These berries are rich in benzoic acid, which has a strong antioxidant effect.

Thanks to their natural preservatives and their high vitamin C content, cranberries also became an essential food for New England sailors in colonial days. No oranges or limes grew in the Northeast, but cranberries grew in abundance and could be taken on sea voyages to ward off scurvy.

Relish Your Cranberries
If pemmican isn't your style, there are still plenty of ways to incorporate cranberries into your diet. Here are a few:

- Try enhancing wild rice with dried cranberries, onions, and orange zest.
- Serve dried cranberries with nuts as finger food at your next party.
- Make a tangy topping for skinless breast of chicken by using chopped fresh or frozen cranberries, diced apple, and chopped walnuts. Melt Monterey Jack cheese over the top.
- When eating out, boost your fruit intake by ordering cranberry juice—or be adventurous and order a more unusual selection, like cranberry juice mixed with grapefruit juice. That way, you get to draw from two color groups at once, plus you get lots of great phytochemicals.
- Sauté green beans with dried cranberries and a little orange zest. Colorful and delicious!

(First three ideas courtesy of Ocean Spray)

Banishing Urinary Tract Infections
What cranberries are best known for today—other than Thanksgiving relish—is warding off urinary tract infections (UTIs). A preventive dose of 10 ounces of cranberry juice a day has long since

passed out of the realm of folk medicine and is well accepted. But why does cranberry juice have this effect? For years, scientists attributed it to the acidity of the juice. But Amy Howell, a research scientist at the Rutgers University Blueberry-Cranberry Research Center, never bought that theory. "If so, then why doesn't lemon juice or grapefruit juice work?" she asks.

Howell and her colleagues discovered the reason. This time it doesn't relate to pigments, although the red anthocyanins in cranberries do have beneficial antioxidant properties. Instead, the reason is a group of larger molecules called *A-linked condensed tannins*. These members of the polyphenolic family act as a sort of Teflon coating to prevent *E. coli* bacteria from adhering to the walls of the bladder and urethra. Exactly how they accomplish that feat is not entirely clear. They could be wrapping themselves around the *E. coli,* so that the bacteria cannot grab onto receptors in the urinary tract lining. Alternatively, the tannins could be blocking the receptors themselves, so that there is no room for the bacteria to dock. However they do it, the result is that the bacteria just slide right on through the body without hanging around to cause infections. "The best part," says Howell, "is that tannins prevent infection without killing the bacteria, so you don't get a buildup of resistance, as you would with antibiotics." Howell recently completed a study comparing various cranberry products and their effectiveness in blocking *E. coli*. "Dried cranberries, or Craisins, were just as effective as the juice per serving," she says. "Cranberry sauces and jellies were sixty to eighty percent as strong."

The only problem with cranberries is that they are not very effective once an infection has actually taken hold. By then, cranberries can only really help if the infection is still in its earliest stages, when the bacteria are only weakly bound to the walls of the urinary tract. As the infection progresses, the bacteria bind more securely, and only antibiotics will knock them out.

Cranberry Toothpaste?

Just as cranberries prevent *E. coli* from sticking to the walls of the urinary tract, they may keep bacteria in the mouth from sticking to teeth and forming dental plaque. That at least was the conclusion of one Israeli study. If cranberries prove as effective in people as they did in that test-tube study, who knows? Maybe one day cranberry extract will be added to toothpaste or mouthwash.

Beyond UTIs

Research out of the University of California, Irvine, suggests that cranberry juice can fight other types of bacteria, too, including staph and salmonella infections. And scientists at Tel Aviv University have found that cranberry extracts can prevent ulcer-causing *Helicobacter pylori* from adhering to the stomach lining—at least in test-tube experiments.

Cranberries may also ward off heart disease through a duo of heart-healthy effects. The red anthocyanin pigments are antioxidants that seem to retard the oxidation of "bad" cholesterol, according to lab tests at the University of Wisconsin-La Crosse. The anthocyanins also appear to reduce platelet clumping in lab tests. That's important because this thins the blood, reducing one's risk of developing heart-attack–inducing clots.

Cranberries might even help prevent breast cancer. Biochemist Najla Guthrie of the University of Western Ontario demonstrated this using three groups of mice. She fed one group a normal, healthy diet. She gave the second group the same diet, but added cranberry juice instead of water to drink. She fed the third group a normal diet supplemented with cranberry "presscake"—that is, cranberries with the juice pressed out.

The results? "The cranberry presscake inhibited the incidence of breast tumors by sixty percent," says Guthrie. "In addition, the spread of tumors to the lungs and lymph nodes was markedly reduced in the cranberry-presscake group." At this early stage, she does not know what compound is causing this effect or how it's doing it. But cranberries do contain cancer-fighting ellagic acid. They also contain one of the most potent cancer-fighting components in tea—a compound with the challenging name *epigallocatechin gallate* (EGCG). "Whatever the active compound is, it's active in small quantities," she says.

Why Are Cranberries So Bitter?

The Pequot Indians referred to cranberries as *i-bimi,* meaning "bitter berry." They weren't kidding. Normally, *The Color Code* frowns on any juice that isn't 100 percent fruit juice, but we have to make an exception here. Pure cranberry juice is a bitter brew. That's because the tannins that make the juice so effective against urinary tract infections are extremely sour. This is hardly surprising. That's exactly why the plant makes them—to be unpleasant enough to repel bugs. The question is: Why do cranberries remain so tart, even after they ripen? After all, most other fruit starts off sour, too, but sweetens as it matures.

The difference is that as most fruit ripens in the wild, it relies on animals to disperse the seeds. This means that the fruit has to tempt animals—and to taste good, it has to be sweet. Cranberries, however, don't need animals to spread their seeds. They grow naturally along the banks of streams, where ripe berries can simply plop into the water and float off to a new location.

POMEGRANATES

Pomegranates at a Glance
- Pigments: anthocyanins (various forms of delphinidin, malvidin, pelargonidin, and cyanidin)
- Other phytochemicals: ellagic acid, ellagitannin, chlorogenic acid, gallic acid, tannins, lignans
- Serving size: 1 medium fruit
- Vitamins and minerals per serving: C (15% of the Daily Value), pantothenic acid (9% DV), potassium (11% DV), iron (3% DV)
- Fiber per serving: 4% DV
- ORAC score: not available

According to ancient Greek mythology, Demeter, the goddess of the grains and the harvest, had a lovely daughter named Persephone. One day, while Persephone was plucking lilies and violets, a chasm opened before her, and Hades, god of the underworld, snatched her away with him to the land of the dead. Lost in grief, Demeter stopped caring for crops. Seeds refused to sprout; harvests withered and died. Demeter finally learned the whereabouts of her daughter and appealed to the god Zeus for assistance in getting Persephone back. Zeus commanded Hades to release the maiden—provided she had eaten nothing while she was in the underworld. But she had. She had eaten some pomegranate seeds that Hades had given her. Therefore, Persephone could return for only part of each year. And so, mythology tells us, the cycle of seasons began. When Persephone departed for the underworld, her mother grieved, flowers withered, and trees shed their leaves. When she returned, Demeter rejoiced, and the fruits of the earth blossomed. Because the pomegranate was associated with Persephone, it came to stand, paradoxically, for both death and fertility.

Of the two, fertility seems much more logical. The most notable feature of the pomegranate is that it is filled with seeds, an obvious sign of fecundity. (The word "pomegranate" itself means "grain-" or "seed-filled apple.") The Babylonians associated the pomegranate's bounty of seeds with resurrection. The Persians believed the seeds would make them invincible in battle. Whether they ensured invincibility or not, pomegranates were an important food. Desert caravans took them on long journeys because they were one of the few fruits that were durable enough to withstand long, hot voyages, and still offer a thirst-quenching juice.

Today, scientists are starting to discern entirely new virtues in pomegranates. The work is preliminary. But researchers in Israel found that in a population of healthy men, pomegranate juice reduced the susceptibility of "bad" cholesterol to oxidation by 43 percent. In the same study, oxidation of cholesterol in mice was reduced even more—by up to 90 percent. But the most dramatic finding was that atherosclerotic lesions in these mice actually shrank by 44 percent. That's right. It didn't just prevent plaques from forming, but also reduced those that were already there!

The reasons are still under investigation. But lipids expert Michael Aviram of the Technion-Israel Institute of Technology, who conducted the study, believes that the anthocyanins and tannins in pomegranates boost levels of an enzyme called *paraoxonase*, which breaks down oxidized cholesterol. Aviram has demonstrated that paraoxonase attacks not only oxidized cholesterol in the bloodstream, but also in atherosclerotic lesions, including fatty streaks, plaques, and atheromas. In a new study, he found that in patients with diseased arteries, just four ounces of pomegranate juice a day for one year actually decreased the size of lesions in their carotid arteries. "We've known that antioxidant chemicals in red wine, ginger, tomatoes, and pomegranates help preserve paraoxonase in the blood," says Aviram. "Now we can see that this not only prevents lesions, but also breaks them down when they form." It's conceivable, he says, that increased consumption of pomegranates may even help atherosclerosis regress naturally, before patients have to resort to angioplasty and bypass surgery.

How Do You Eat Pomegranates?

Admittedly, the pomegranate at first appears unassailable—a tough armor on the outside and a mass of seeds on the inside. The easiest way to serve pomegranates is to take a knife and deeply score the fruit several times from top to bottom, like longitude lines. Then break the fruit apart along these lines and pull out the clusters of seeds. Each seed is coated in a fleshy red pulp. The seeds may be eaten plain or used to top a tasty spinach-pear salad. Another great option is to buy concentrated pomegranate juice at the health food store. Then add a spoonful or two to a glass of orange juice for a simple treat that tastes surprisingly like apricot nectar.

BEETS

Beets at a Glance

- Pigments: betacyanins (mainly betanin), betaxanthins
- Other phytochemicals: betaine, farnesol, salicylic acid, saponins
- Serving size: half a cup
- Vitamins and minerals per serving: C (5% of the Daily Value), folate (17% DV), potassium (8% DV), magnesium (5% DV), iron (4% DV)
- Fiber per serving: 7% DV
- ORAC score: 840

As anyone who's cooked beets knows, they can be messy. The reason is the rich red pigments that tend to leach out into the sour cream, onto your hands, and all over your apron. In colonial times, beet dye was used to tint icing and to make pancakes pink. If you do not, however, fancy a pink kitchen, then bake, steam, or boil the beets with their tough outer skin intact. Do not remove the root ends until the beets have been cooked and transferred to a separate bowl. Some chefs wear plastic gloves to peel cooked beets.

For a food that's such a rich red, it may come as a surprise that beets have no anthocyanins at all. Their color comes instead from an unusual group of red pigments called *betacyanins,* which also color the beautiful tropical plant bougainvillea. Betacyanins have not been well studied. But researchers suspect that they may prove to be potent cancer fighters, particularly the natural dye *betanin.* In the 1950s, Dr. Alexander Ferenczi in Hungary treated inoperable cancer patients with organic beet juice and grated raw beets. In 21 out of 22 patients, he saw varying degrees of tumor regression and weight gain. In recent years, Govind Kapadia, professor of biomedicinal chemistry at Howard University, has found beet extract to be a "profound" inhibitor of skin, lung, and liver tumors in mice. "We assume it's the red pigments that are having this effect, but that remains to be proven," says Kapadia. Still, the evidence is convincing enough to have launched an alternative practice in Germany, Hungary, and Brazil using beet juice to help cancer patients. Other alternative practitioners use beet juice to treat infections and eliminate parasites.

Beets also contain an unusual substance called *betaine* that's found in few other foods. A colorless crystal, betaine is important because it plays a role in detoxifying homocysteine, a troublesome amino acid that has been implicated in heart disease. Normally, vitamins B_{12} and folate join forces to rid the body of excess homocysteine. But if there is not enough of these, then betaine becomes the pinch hitter and does the job. "It's considered a salvage mechanism," says Teodoro Bottiglieri, director of neuropharmacology at Baylor University's Institute for Metabolic Diseases. "When things get desperate, then betaine kicks in."

Healthy Monks

Like many other fresh fruits and vegetables—and especially herbs and spices—beets contain salicylic acid, a close relative of aspirin (acetylsalicylic acid). A recent study in Scotland compared Buddhist monks with a group of meat eaters. The vegetarian monks had significantly higher levels of salicylic acid in their blood than the nonvegetarians. In some cases, they had as much as patients who take aspirin daily. Salicylic acid does not thin the blood, as aspirin does. But because it has anti-inflammatory properties, the scientists speculated that salicylic acid might account, in part, for the health-promoting effects of fruit and vegetables. Stay tuned.

APPLES

Apples at a Glance
- Pigments: anthocyanins (various forms of cyanidin and malvidin), beta-carotene
- Other phytochemicals: quercetin, myricetin, rutin, ferulic acid, glucaric acid, D-glucaric acid
- Serving size: one medium apple
- Vitamins and minerals per serving: A (2% of the Daily Value), C (13% DV), potassium (5% DV), copper (3% DV), iron (2% DV)
- Fiber: 15% DV
- ORAC score: 218

Americans have had a love affair with apples ever since John Chapman—better known as Johnny Appleseed—traveled the country in the early 1800s, planting apple seeds along the way. As pioneers moved west, planting apple trees was a sign that they intended to settle in a new locale. Some land companies even required settlers to plant apple orchards in order to claim a parcel of land. Apples are as American as, well, apple pie. And that's not even taking into account their supposed health benefits. The saying "An apple a day keeps the doctor away" is just the modern version of an older saying from Devonshire, England, in the 1500s: "Ate an apfel avore gwain to bed. Makes the doctor beg his bread."

Do apples really deserve all this acclaim? They are obviously not the best source of pigments. Except for a thin skin, they're white throughout. And did you ever wonder why apples float when you bob for them? It's because 25 percent of their volume is air. They're not the best source of vitamins or minerals, either. They don't contain large amounts of any of them.

That's three strikes, but apples are not out. Here's why. If you eat apples *with the skin*, you tap into an important reserve of flavonoids, including *quercetin*. In lab studies, quercetin shows numerous health benefits. It is a strong antioxidant that can "quench" a particularly damaging free radical called singlet oxygen. It can kill viruses such as herpes simplex and enhance the fighting capability of other antiviral compounds. And together with other flavonoids, it fights inflammation. That's why it's used clinically to alleviate inflammatory problems, including gout, pancreatitis, and prostatitis. It's also used to treat allergic conditions such as asthma, hay fever, and hives. In a new study, Sarah Lewis at the Univeristy of Nottingham in England examined the eating habits of 2,633 adults and correlated them with wheezing, asthma, and lung capacity. Those with the healthiest lungs ate apples at least five times a week and tomatoes three times a week.

Of all the fruits, apples (both red and green) contain the highest levels of quercetin. Given quercetin's antioxidant and anti-inflammatory strength, this flavonoid may be the reason why apples are connected with heart health. One study of 804 elderly Dutch men examined their intakes of 49 foods, then followed the men for 10 years to see how many had fatal or non-fatal heart attacks. Those men who ate the most flavonoids—in particular, quercetin—had 53 percent fewer fatal heart attacks than those who ate the least. Three foods stood out—tea, onions, and apples, in that order.

Apples May Reduce Cancer Risk

Apples may also reduce cancer risk. A Finnish study of 9,959 men and women found that those who ate the most flavonoid-rich foods decreased their rates of all tumors, especially lung cancer. Over the 24 years of the study, they slashed their risks of lung cancer by half. And one food in particular seemed to do the trick—apples. Similarly, a Hawaiian study found less lung cancer among those who dined on onions and apples.

Quercetin appears to be one of the main reasons for these anti-carcinogenic effects. Scientists have found that it possesses an impressive arsenal of cancer-fighting strategies. For example, it can inhibit the growth of malignant cells and cause abnormal cells to self-destruct, through apoptosis. And according to a new study from the Mayo Clinic, it has one more potent effect. In prostate tumor cells in the lab, it restricts the cells' production of androgen receptors. That's important because overstimulation of those receptors by the male hormones appears to drive the development of prostate cancer.

But researchers emphasize that you couldn't get all the benefits of apples from a simple quercetin supplement. Although quercetin appears to be one of the most potent flavonoids in apples, it is much more powerful when combined with the fruit's other natural compounds, as Mother Nature conveniently packaged them. Rui Hai Liu, who teaches food science at Cornell University, demonstrated this by putting human cancer cells into special containers with all the nutrients they would need to grow. Then he added either quercetin or whole-apple extract from Red Delicious apples. The idea was to see whether either substance could inhibit the growth of the cancer cells. Both did. But the whole-apple extract outperformed the quercetin by a long shot.

Much of that health-promoting power comes from the peel. In a second test-tube experiment with liver cancer cells, Liu added extracts from either peeled or unpeeled Red Delicious apples. Guess which worked the best? Apples with the peels on were 50 percent better at stopping cancer-cell proliferation. "The good phytochemicals are in the skin," says Liu. That goes for both red and green apples.

Eat an Apple a Day

If your kids refuse to eat apple skins, do not despair. At least they will be getting fiber. Eighty percent of the fiber in apples is in the white flesh of the fruit.

Fiber comes in two varieties—soluble and insoluble. Neither one is absorbed from the digestive tract into the bloodstream. But both are valuable.

The flesh of apples contains soluble fiber, most of it in a form called *pectin*. This is the same stuff that's used to thicken jellies. Just as it thickens strawberry jam, pectin bulks up in the stomach, making you feel full. At the same time, it temporarily binds sugars, so that they don't rush into the bloodstream at once. Pectin releases these sugars gradually, keeping blood sugar levels steady.

Pectin's main claim to dietary fame, however, is that it lowers cholesterol. In one study, 25 men drank 20 ounces of unfiltered, fiber-supplemented apple juice every day for six weeks. On average, the apple fiber lowered their total cholesterol by 10 percent—and LDL cholesterol by 14 percent. The reason seems to be that pectin acts as a giant sponge, sopping up cholesterol and bile acids in the digestive tract. Because the body can't digest fiber, the pectin passes right on through the system, taking cholesterol along with it! In a recent Finnish study of 9,208 men and women, those who ate apples cut their risk of stroke by 40 percent over a 28-year period. The effect was apparently not due to the quercetin. Perhaps it was the fiber.

If you eat the peel along with the apple, you get even more fiber, particularly *in*soluble fiber (better known as roughage). True to the name, insoluble fiber does not dissolve in water. Nor does the body absorb it. Its virtue lies in the fact that it adds bulk to the stool and eases it on out, helping to prevent such conditions as irritable bowel syndrome and diverticulosis.

QUICK 'N' EASY

Eating right can be a challenge in today's society—if for no other reason than lack of time. As the bumper sticker says: "If a woman's place is in the home, why am I always in my car?" But there's no excuse for skimping on apples. They're nature's version of fast food. Not to compare apples to oranges, but let's face it, nothing could be simpler than polishing up an apple and sinking your teeth into it. The best way to encourage yourself to eat these fruits is to keep some on hand for snacks. If they're readily available, you're more likely to reach for them when the munchies strike.

To boost your consumption even more, make an autumn visit to a farm where you and your family can enjoy apple picking. Almost any food tastes better fresh-picked, especially when you're the one who's picked it. And the bushel you bring home will encourage you to get creative with new ways to eat apples. Here are some ideas:

> - Top whole-wheat French toast with sliced apples and a sprinkle of cinnamon.
> - Stuff baked apples with dried apricots, orange zest, orange juice, and brown sugar.
> - Cut up apple chunks to dip into a fondue made with reduced-fat cheese.
> - Make your own applesauce. Be sure to include lemon for a zestier flavor and the apple skins to boost your flavonoids.
>
> (NOTE: First two ideas courtesy of the Washington Apple Commission)

RED ONIONS

Red Onions at a Glance
- Pigments: anthocyanins (various forms of cyanidin and pelargonidin)
- Other phytochemicals: quercetin, kaempferol, allicin, alliin, diallyl disulfide, caffeic acid, ferulic acid, fructooligosaccharides
- Serving size: half a cup
- Vitamins and minerals per serving: C (8% of the Daily Value), B_6 (5% DV), folate (4% DV), thiamin (2% DV), potassium (4% DV), calcium (2% DV)
- Fiber per serving: 6% DV
- ORAC score: 450 (yellow onions; not available for red onions)

Onions are circles within circles. Peel back one layer, and you find another, and yet another. Perhaps because of this structure, many people in the ancient world associated onions with eternal life. But onions were known to offer plenty of benefits for the living, too. An Egyptian papyrus described them as a tonic for the blood. Pliny the Elder, who lived in Pompeii, wrote that onions were grown in that city and used to heal sores, toothaches, and dysentery. As recently as 1864, General Ulysses S. Grant declared during the American Civil War: "I will not move my army without onions!" He believed that onions would help keep his men healthy in the swampy southern climate. He may have been right. Just as onions peel back layer after layer, their benefits seem to unfold one after another, revealing reason upon reason to eat the tasty bulbs.

"Rocket Fuel" for Humans

The most notable reason for eating onions—other than flavor enhancement—is to tap into the *organosulfur* compounds, which are found exclusively in onions and their relatives, including garlic, leeks, chives, and scallions. The organosulfur compounds work sort of like the liquid rocket fuel that helps propel the space shuttle. The components of the liquid fuel are kept in two separate compartments. Only at launch are they combined, with explosive effects. In the same way, the organosulfur components in onions— amino acids and sulfoxides—are separated by a membrane. But when an insect starts to nibble or a chef's knife slices through, it disrupts the membranes, allowing the compounds to mix, forming pungent, tear-inducing compounds. These compounds not only repel insects and add flavor but also appear to ward off cancer, at least in lab animals. "We've found the sulfur compounds in garlic and onions very promising for colon, esophagus, and breast cancer," says Michael Wargovich, director of basic research at the South Carolina Cancer Center.

These compounds may also turn out to be potent heart medicine. Irwin Goldman, associate professor of horticulture at the University of Wisconsin in Madison, has found that they help thin the blood and prevent unwanted clotting. "When we feed animals pungent raw onions, it has a marked effect on blood thinning," says Goldman. "In test tube work, the organosulfur compounds are more potent than aspirin."

For reasons that aren't clear, onions also improve the ratio of "good" to "bad" cholesterol in the blood. Dr. Victor Gurewich at Harvard Medical School performed a series of experiments in the mid-1980s, showing that consumption of onions could raise beneficial HDL by as much as 30 percent. Total cholesterol remained the same. "The equivalent of one medium onion a day was sufficient," says Gurewich. "Raw onions were more effective than cooked." Gurewich never identified exactly which components of onions had this effect, but he did note that the active compounds were in the volatile, fume-producing portion. That points toward the organosulfur compounds.

The Ultimate Disease-Fighting Onion

All onions—white, yellow, and red—contain the organosulfur compounds in varying amounts. (The more pungent the bulb, the more organosulfur compounds it contains.) But if you eat either yellow or red onions, you also get the flavonoid quercetin. Go one better and buy red onions, and you may have the ultimate onion for disease protection, particularly if it's a pungent one. That's because red onions contain organosulfur compounds, quercetin, *and* anthocyanin pigments. "And red onions are super high in quercetin, because it's related to the anthocyanins," says Irwin Goldman.

This quercetin could help chip away at both cancer and heart disease. A study at the University of Hawaii assessed 582 patients with lung cancer and matched them against cancer-free controls. Those who ate the most onions reduced their lung cancer risk by 50 percent; those who ate the most apples, by 40 percent. The onion crowd had especially low levels of a type of lung cancer called squamous cell carcinoma. In addition, studies show that onions are even better heart protectors than apples, probably because onions contain larger quantities of flavonoids, including quercetin. These flavonoids function as antioxidants, helping to fight the oxidation of "bad" cholesterol—and also work as anti-inflammatories. In effect, you get two benefits for the price of one.

Boning Up on Onions

When most of us think about preventing osteoporosis, we think of calcium-rich, vitamin-D-fortified milk. Maybe we should think of onions, too. The research is highly preliminary, but when researchers at the University of Bern in Switzerland fed male rats 1 gram of powdered onion every day for a month, it boosted the mineral content of their bones by over 17 percent and increased bone thickness by almost 15 percent. In fact, onion therapy was slightly more effective than osteoporosis drugs based on calcitonin!

Since osteoporosis poses the greatest risk for postmenopausal women, the researchers also tried the same experiment in female rats who had their ovaries removed to mimic menopause. The consequent drop in bone-protecting estrogen caused the rats to suffer bone loss of 32 percent. This effect, however, could be drastically reduced by adding onion to the animals' diets. Those who were given the most onion had 25 percent less bone loss than those who received none. If the same holds true for humans, the researchers concluded, "then including an appropriate amount of these vegetables in the daily diet could be an effective and inexpensive way to decrease the incidence of osteoporosis."

QUICK 'N' EASY

For a quick, refreshing summer salad, try this version of an Italian panzanella.

Chop one large tomato, one medium cucumber, and one small red onion. Toss them in a bowl with a dressing of olive oil and balsamic vinegar. Add your favorite salad seasonings and fresh chopped basil.

Don't Cry Over Your Onions

An eleventh-century riddle includes the following clue: "No one suffers at my hands except for my slayer." The answer, of course, is an onion. Anyone who's ever felt their eyes itch, sting, and water while chopping an onion will not dispute that. Fortunately, there are ways to take the sting out of onions. The simplest is to chill the onions first. That makes the offensive compounds less volatile. Another solution is to grasp a piece of bread between your teeth and hold it there while chopping. As the fumes rise, they will be absorbed by the bread before reaching your eyes. For a third option, try rinsing your knife under cold water before beginning to chop.

ORANGE-YELLOW

"Of all our foods, corn most resembles woman, with an enticing aroma, silky locks, and nourishment for civilizations."

—Anonymous

A WHIFF OF SPRING AIR, the warble of songbirds, tender spring green buds . . . the inevitable April showers. As the first gentle drops begin to fall, what could be more comforting than a bright yellow raincoat? Yellow and orange are perhaps the ultimate comfort colors. Just think of the things they represent— warm summer sunshine, autumn leaves, cozy fires, fields of golden grain. Just as you pull your raincoat close around you, surround yourself with orange and yellow foods. They mean protection.

CARROTS

Carrots at a Glance
- Pigments: alpha-carotene, beta-carotene, beta-cryptoxanthin, lutein, lycopene
- Other phytochemicals: apigenin, pinene, terpinene, terpineol, d-limonene, myricetin, caffeic acid, p-coumaric acid, chlorogenic acid
- Serving size: one medium carrot
- Vitamins and minerals per serving: A (330% of the Daily Value), C (12% DV), potassium (7% DV), calcium (2% DV)
- Fiber per serving: 12% DV
- ORAC score: 207

One day, perhaps 2,000 years ago, someone in Afghanistan noticed that the thick roots of a feathery green weed had a sweet taste. Over the years, Afghans began cultivating this weed, the carrot. So did the Indians, Chinese, Japanese, and eventually the Europeans. Who could resist a vegetable that was both delicious and easy to store through the cold winter months? When carrots finally arrived in England around Elizabethan times, this new plant became a great curiosity. In 1599, Richard Gardiner wrote in his horticultural manual, "Sowe carrots in your gardens, and humbly praise God for them, as for a singular and great blessing." Not only did they taste good, but they also intrigued ladies and gentlemen alike with their delicate green foliage. Women plucked off sprigs and wore them as decorations in their hats and hair.

Today, we think of carrots as orange. But that wasn't always the case. The first carrots came in a broad palette of colors, including red, yellow, and purple. In fact, no one had ever heard of an orange carrot until some pale orange ones were bred in the Netherlands in the 1700s. For reasons that remain obscure, orange carrots became the standard. But other hues still exist. At least one seed company in the United States peddles seeds for scarlet carrots. A delicious purple carrot called the Beta Sweet can be purchased in specialty groceries. And farmers occasionally pluck what they expect to be an orange carrot from the ground, only to find that it is either partly or wholly maroon. (The red-tinged ones never make it to market, but are used to feed farm animals.)

Could You Learn to Love a Purple Carrot?

Admittedly, the Beta Sweet carrot wouldn't win any beauty contests. The outside is a deep purple verging on black. At first glance, it looks as if it must have been stricken by some terrible blight. But skim off the dull surface, and underneath it glistens with a rich, succulent red-purple sheen. Slice it crosswise, and inside the thick purple layer you'll find a bright orange core. Clearly, this is no ordinary carrot. Even its taste is distinctive—more like an apple than a carrot, with a sweet, moist crunch.

How did such an unusual specimen come to be? Leonard Pike, director of the Vegetable and Fruit Improvement Center at Texas A&M University, developed the hybrid after abandoning earlier plans to breed a novelty carrot in maroon and white—the school colors of Texas A&M. Research on the health benefits of anthocyanins and carotenoids persuaded him to get serious, he says, and to maximize the colors in his new carrot. Good plan! The Beta Sweet lets you cover two color groups at once—purple and orange—and fulfill 170 percent of your daily vitamin A need, too. As an added bonus, it gives you 6 percent of your daily iron requirement.

One tip: Cut off the leafy green tops, as you would with any carrots before storing them. Otherwise, the greens will draw out moisture, and the carrots will wilt faster.

What's Up, Doc?

Carrots could be the original health food. Again and again, they turn up in studies as major disease fighters. For example:

- When the World Cancer Research Fund reviewed 206 human studies, carrots consistently emerged as one of the top cancer-fighting foods, along with green vegetables, tomatoes, and crucifers (such as broccoli, cabbage, and cauliflower).
- Carrots also appear to reduce the risk of stroke. Perhaps the most dramatic finding came out of the Nurses' Health Study in 1993. JoAnn Manson and her colleagues at Harvard tracked 87,000 nurses for eight years. Those who ate just five large carrots a week lowered their risk of stroke by 68 percent, compared with those who ate only one carrot a month or none at all!
- Carrots lower cholesterol levels, too, thanks in part to their fiber content. A classic study in Great Britain showed that by munching on two large carrots a day for three weeks, participants reduced their cholesterol levels by 11 percent. That's as much as patients often achieve with medication.

In fact, no one has documented any adverse effects at all from eating carrots—except one minor inconvenience. If you eat a lot of them, your body may store the extra beta-carotene in your skin, giving it a yellow-orange tinge (common in infants and young children, since puréed carrots are a popular baby food). Not to worry.

This so-called carotenemia is a harmless condition that will go away shortly after your carrot consumption returns to normal.

Don't Worry About the Sugar

Certain popular diets urge people to avoid carrots because they contain a lot of natural sugar. We couldn't disagree more strongly with that advice. Although carrots contain more sugar than any vegetable except beets, the fiber in carrots prevents this sugar from rushing into the bloodstream and causing insulin spikes, as the fearmongers would have it. Skip carrots, and you'll miss out on a prime source of beta-carotene and other health-promoting phytonutrients. So munch away. A bag of organic baby carrots makes a delicious—and healthful—snack.

Vitamin A: "Tremendously Wonderful"

One of the major health-promoting compounds in carrots is unquestionably the orange pigment *beta-carotene*. Beta-carotene has garnered a lot of publicity in recent years as an antioxidant. But it is even more essential to the body for another reason. "Beta-carotene may not be a biologically important antioxidant, but it's a major source of vitamin A," says nutrition scientist Cheryl Rock of the University of California, San Diego. "And vitamin A does tremendously wonderful things."

Although some effects of vitamin A are well known, others are still being discovered. As scientists have known for decades, the vitamin is crucial for eyesight—so important that vitamin A was given the chemical name "retinol," after the retina, the thin layer of light-sensitive cells in the back of the eyeball that enables us to see. More recently, researchers have learned that the vitamin also plays a critical role in maintaining the immune system, the skin, and the so-called epithelial cells that line every organ. That's important, because 85 percent of cancers start in these cells.

Preliminary work has indicated that vitamin A is even crucial to learning and memory. Ronald Evans, professor of gene expression at the Salk Institute for Biological Studies, has found that the hippocampus—the area of the brain that specializes in memory formation—cannot work properly without it. When he deprived mice of vitamin A, they were unable to perform a memory task that should have grown easier with repetition. Normally, by the fifth time through, the average mouse has no trouble with the test. But for the mice without vitamin A in their diets, "It was as if they'd never tried it before," says Evans. "To the outside world, they look normal. They swim, they eat, they do most things normally. But they can't learn." When he put the animals back on vitamin A, they began learning again. That doesn't mean that eating extra carrots will improve your memory—but it does suggest that if you aren't getting enough vitamin A, as is often the case in developing countries, your ability to learn and remember may be impaired.

"Value Added"

After all this powerful vitamin A activity, anything beta-carotene can accomplish as an antioxidant is just icing on the carrot cake, so to speak. "It's value added," says Rock. But how much value? Scientists really don't know. According to Lester Packer, a leading authority on antioxidants, beta-carotene is not one of the first-line antioxidants in the body. Those honors go to vitamins C and E, plus three substances that the body itself produces—alpha-lipoic acid, coenzyme Q10, and glutathione. In fact, beta-carotene seems exceptionally weak at some of the classic functions of antioxidants, such as fighting heart disease.

We know that it does function as an antioxidant at some level, because pharmaceutical-grade beta-carotene beadlets are the FDA-approved treatment of choice for a rare skin disease involving unusual levels of free-radical damage. "People with this disease can develop severe pain and burning sensations in sun-exposed skin after only brief exposures to sunlight," says Dr. Micheline Mathews-Roth of Harvard Medical School. Beta-carotene is the antioxidant that absorbs those free radicals and lets susceptible individuals lead almost normal lives.

Antioxidant capacity may also account for beta-carotene's apparent ability to boost the activity of tumor-scavenging cells known as natural-killer cells. A study of 59 physicians in Boston found that natural-killer–cell activity was much higher in elderly men who had taken beta-carotene supplements for 10 years than in those who had not. "Oxidative stress damages natural-killer cells in ways that may affect the cells' activity," says Simin Meydani, professor of nutrition and immunology at Tufts and one of the researchers who conducted the study. Other studies have achieved even better immune enhancement using fruit and vegetable extracts that contained a mixture of the major carotenoids.

A Cellular Hearing Aid

Even if beta-carotene isn't a first-line antioxidant, it has other remarkable properties. For example, it stimulates enzymes that repair damaged DNA. In a German study of 23 healthy men, beta-carotene–rich carrot juice and lycopene-rich tomato juice were both effective at this task. But beta-carotene doesn't indiscriminately activate all enzymes. On the contrary, it inhibits the rate-limiting enzyme in cholesterol synthesis. That's why studies show that beta-carotene (and lycopene, too) can help reduce cholesterol.

Beta-carotene also aids a type of cellular communication that can help stifle malignancies. Cells sometimes become alarmed by abnormal replication in a neighboring cell and send it an urgent message—*stop dividing*. If the aberrant cell can't "hear" the message, it can't heed it. But beta-carotene aids cellular "hearing" by switching on a gene that produces tiny entrances into the cell for diminutive messengers from neighboring cells. (Larger messengers aren't allowed in, but have to dock in special receptors on the cell's surface.) Because these same tiny doorways allow message-bearing molecules out, they also aid cellular "talking" as well as "hearing."

Cell biologist John Bertram at the Cancer Research Center of the University of Hawaii has found that all the major dietary carotenoids—including lycopene, lutein, and beta-cryptoxanthin—aid these cellular communications. But beta-carotene does it better than any of the others. Bertram has set up cell cultures where he can literally see cellular communications taking place under the microscope. He does this by tagging messenger molecules with fluorescent compounds and then watching them move from one cell to the next. If the cells aren't "talking" to one another, the tagged molecule stays in one place. If the communications are functioning smoothly, the fluorescent dot moves easily through the group of cells. "You can actually see it happening in real time," Bertram says. "When graduate students see it for the first time, they gasp in amazement."

Healthier Carrots

The average carrot today has more beta-carotene in it than it did a generation ago. That's because scientists have been deliberately crossbreeding them to produce hybrids with higher beta-carotene contents. According to Philipp Simon, professor of horticulture at University of Wisconsin in Madison, the amount of beta-carotene in carrots has increased by about 60 percent over the last 20 years. "The color is more intense, but not so striking that you'll be put off," he says. In fact, packagers often try to make carrots look even more colorful by printing thin red stripes across the plastic bag.

Shifting Colors

The colors of pigments can vary according to their concentrations. Red anthocyanins, for example, can appear dark purple or even black if they are dense enough, as in the Beta Sweet carrot.

Similarly, a number of carotenoids appear yellow in low concentrations, but orange at greater densities. For example, alpha- and beta-carotene look orange in carrots, where they are densely packed. But in summer squash, where beta-carotene and lutein are more sparsely distributed, they produce a lighter yellow tint.

That's a powerful reason to fortify your diet with the more intensely colored fruits and vegetables. You get greater levels of health-promoting pigments.

More Reasons to Munch a Bunch

With all the hoopla over beta-carotene, we tend to forget that carrots also contain a hearty brew of other cancer-fighting phytochemicals. *Alpha-carotene,* a close relative of beta-carotene, is one. In a series of Japanese lab studies, it was ten times more effective than beta-carotene at stopping proliferation of human cancer cells. And in a recent follow-up study of 124,207 nurses and health professionals, Harvard researchers found that nonsmokers who consumed the most alpha-carotene–rich foods reduced their risk of lung cancer by a whopping 63 percent. (When smokers were added into the mix, the most potent effect came from a combination of all six major carotenoids—alpha-and beta-carotene, lycopene, beta-cryptoxanthin, lutein, and zeaxanthin.) Because we eat so many carrots, they supply more than half the alpha-carotene in our diets.

It's not only the pigments in carrots that fight disease. So do the compounds that impart flavor. One of them is a terpenoid called *terpineol*. But carrots don't produce terpineol to create a pleasant taste for humans. They make it to fight fungi. That's because terpineol interferes with the production of substances that fungi require in order to grow. By coincidence, cancer cells need the very same substances, so terpineol helps fight tumors, too. It also encourages something called *cell cycle arrest* in tumors. "Cells have to divide in order to multiply," says Charles Elson, professor of nutritional sciences at the University of Wisconsin College of Agriculture and Life Sciences. "If they can't complete the division process, they die a slow death."

Carrots also contain a flavone called *apigenin*, which has anti-bacterial, antihistaminic, anti-inflammatory, antioxidant, antitumor, and sun-protective properties, according to a USDA database. Diane Birt at Iowa State University has studied its effects on laboratory animals and human cancer cells for 15 years. Her findings: Like terpineol, apigenin causes cell cycle arrest in tumor cells. If given in sufficient quantities, it stops cell replication in its tracks.

Bet on Carrots Rather Than Supplements

With all these cancer-busting phytochemicals, it's no wonder that carrots turn up repeatedly in studies as potent cancer-fighting foods. Beta-carotene clearly contributes to the effect. Yet in two important trials, beta-carotene supplements actually *increased* lung cancer rates in heavy smokers. Does that mean that beta-carotene isn't good for us after all? No way. There are several possible explanations.

Many scientists have speculated that beta-carotene pills were given too late to help these high-risk patients, who may already have had undetected tumors at the start of the trial.

Others point out that beta-carotene is just one of many cancer-crushing compounds in carrots. If you take beta-carotene pills alone, you're missing out on the rest. "A single carotenoid probably won't be a magic bullet for such a complex situation as cancer," says Frederick Khachik, a carotenoids expert and organic chemist at the University of Maryland. Excessive doses of beta-carotene may even block the absorption of other, equally important carotenoids such as alpha-carotene.

Finally, beta-carotene appears to behave differently at very high supplemental doses than it does when consumed in foods. (The two trials gave participants 20 or 30 milligrams of beta-carotene a day—on top of their normal daily intake of approximately 1.5 to 3 milligrams from food.) "In excessive doses, virtually all antioxidants can behave as pro-oxidants," says Robert Russell, associate director of the Human Nutrition Research Center on Aging at Tufts. "Instead of inhibiting cancer, they may promote it." Rest assured, you cannot get harmful doses from foods, no matter how many carrots you eat. You can't even overdose on a one-a-day supplement, so far as anyone knows. (Moreover, one-a-days have been shown to help reduce a number of potentially harmful deficiencies.) But fistfuls of pills could be a different matter. Bottom line: If you smoke, don't count on beta-carotene tablets to save you.

By the way, beta-carotene is not the only nutrient that has proven disappointing when tested in isolation. Recent studies with supplements of vitamin E, vitamin C, and fiber have also failed to achieve the desired results. So if you're gulping down pills to compensate for a diet of bacon and donuts, consider switching to a colorful, semi-vegetarian diet instead. That's the only way to take advantage of the full spectrum of health-giving compounds in fruits and vegetables.

QUICK 'N' EASY

One of the easiest possible ways to boost your vegetable intake is to buy packages of organic baby carrots—prepeeled, prewashed. All you do is open the package and pop them into your mouth for a naturally sweet, delicious snack—with few calories and virtually no fat.

SWEET POTATOES

Sweet Potatoes at a Glance
- Pigments: beta-carotene
- Other phytochemicals: caffeic acid, chlorogenic acid, quercetin
- Serving size: one medium sweet potato
- Vitamins and minerals per serving (baked with the skin): A (498% of the Daily Value), C (47% DV), E (26% DV), thiamin (10% DV), B_6 (14% DV), riboflavin (8% DV), folate (7% DV), B_{12} (7% DV), manganese (32% DV), copper (12% DV), potassium (11% DV), magnesium (6% DV), phosphorus (6% DV), iron (3% DV)
- Fiber per serving: 14% DV
- ORAC score: 301

Today, ginseng enjoys a reputation as an aphrodisiac. But in Shakespeare's day, one of the most popular aphrodisiacs was sweet potatoes. In 1586, Thomas Dawson published a recipe for a sweet potato tart "that is a courage to man or woman." (Everybody knew what "courage" meant in those days, as in the refrain of the old English song, "My husband's got no courage in him, o dear-o.") About the same time, English herbalist John Gerard wrote that sweet potatoes "comfort, nourish, and strengthen the body, vehemently procuring bodily lust." Think about *that* at your next Thanksgiving dinner. Or maybe it's better not to.

Despite these references, sweet potatoes go much further back in history than Shakespeare's time. Archeologists have found the remains of sweet potatoes in Incan and pre-Incan ruins in Peru, dating back thousands of years. When Columbus landed in the New World in 1492, he was apparently intrigued by the delicious vegetable. According to his ship's log, he took some sweet potatoes back to Spain with him. As it turned out, though, sweet potatoes grew particularly well in the American South and became an integral part of southern cooking. "As recently as 50 to 60 years ago, every homestead in rural North Carolina had its own sweet potato patch," says Sue Johnson-Langdon, executive director of the North Carolina SweetPotato (sic) Commission. Now sweet potatoes seem poised to make a major leap onto the national dinner plate, and not just at Thanksgiving. Once regarded as poor man's food, they are now part of the "nouveau soul" or "upscale Gullah" cuisine. In 1995, the sweet potato was declared the official state vegetable of North Carolina.

Good move! Sweet potatoes boast more beta-carotene than any other vegetable, including carrots. They are also one of the few good sources of vitamin E that isn't loaded with fat. The Center for Science in the Public Interest assigned points to 58 vegetables based on their contents of seven nutrients—vitamins A, C, folate, iron, copper, calcium, and fiber. The sweet potato finished first, with a stunning score of 582. Its nearest competitor, the carrot, was nearly 150 points down the list, at 434. The lowly baked potato mustered only 114.

Sweet Potatoes Help Fight the Viral War

How can you lose with a food so rich in nutrients? In addition to all the vitamins, minerals, and fiber, sweet potatoes also contain phytochemicals, such as quercetin and chlorogenic acid, that fight cancer.

In addition, they contain immune-boosting carotenoids. In one small but revealing study, USDA immunologist Tim Kramer had 12 volunteers lunch on kale and sweet potatoes every day for three weeks, with tomato juice to wash it down. These foods ensured high levels of three major carotenoids—beta-carotene (in sweet potatoes), lycopene (in tomato juice), and lutein (in kale). The results? After three weeks, the volunteers had a stunning 33 percent increase in immune response as measured by the ability of their T-cells to multiply. The ability to multiply rapidly is important because the body doesn't keep lots of extra T-cells around for emergencies. Instead, it orders them up on an as-needed basis to fight off viral invaders, just as an army mobilizes its production lines when it gears up for war. Only by producing enough T-cells can the body win the viral war. Carotenoids help the T-cell production lines respond to the threat.

Sweet Potatoes Are Not Potatoes—or Yams, Either

It would be logical to assume that sweet potatoes are a type of potato. But only the name is the same—and the fact that both grow underground. Beyond that, the two vegetables are completely unrelated. Here are some of the differences:

- Sweet potatoes are members of the morning glory family. Potatoes are kin to deadly nightshade.
- Sweet potatoes are roots. By contrast, potatoes are tubers, which are a swollen part of the stem that grows beneath the soil.
- Sweet potatoes are also two-and-a-half times denser than plain spuds, and they're loaded with beta-carotene, which is lacking in white potatoes.

Speaking of identities, sweet potatoes are not yams, either. Although the words "yam" and "sweet potato" are used interchangeably in this country, a true yam comes from yet another botanical family, the lily. Real yams are mainly found overseas in Africa or the Caribbean. They are less flavorful and drier in texture than the sweet potato, and they're also lower in beta-carotene.

YELLOW POTATOES

Although we think of potatoes as white, they come in a stunning array of colors. "When you go to markets in the Andes, you can find potatoes whose flesh is red, orange, yellow, purple, or blue," says Charles Brown, a research geneticist with the USDA's Agricultural Research Service in Prosser, Washington. "The International Potato Center in Lima, Peru, has collected more than two thousand varieties." Many of these colorful strains have greater health benefits than plain white spuds, thanks to their pigments. For example, Brown has used crossbreeding techniques to create an intense red-and-purple–fleshed potato with a nutty flavor and high levels of anthocyanins. Some dark yellow and orange potatoes, he says, are high in the carotenoid zeaxanthin, which helps fight certain eye diseases. (The popular Yukon Gold potatoes, being lighter

> ## QUICK 'N' EASY
>
> Sweet potatoes are so delicious, they're almost decadent. "Just watch a sweet potato bake," says Sue Johnson-Langdon of the North Carolina SweetPotato Commission. "It will ooze syrup. It will soften and caramelize on its own, without a drop of sugar or butter."
>
> If you're pressed for time and don't want to wait 40 to 50 minutes to bake a sweet potato, try microwaving it instead. Just prick the skin several times and microwave for four to six minutes on high power. (For best results, use potatoes that do not vary much in width between the middle and ends.) Or try sweet potatoes raw, as crudités with dips.
>
> If you have more time, Johnson-Langdon recommends roasting sweet potato slices with olive oil, fresh rosemary, pine nuts, and garlic (recipe, page 271) or making a tasty black bean salad with roasted red peppers, ripe papaya, watercress, purple onion, and chili powder (page 245).

in color, contain only small amounts of lutein and zeaxanthin.) If you can get colorful compounds as a bonus in potatoes, why not?

Even pale white spuds are an excellent food, however. Critics carp that they are "just a starch." But plain white potatoes pack a powerhouse of vitamins and minerals. Take a look:

- Phytochemicals: caffeic acid, chlorogenic acid, ferulic acid, alpha-lipoic acid, glutathione
- Serving size: one medium potato
- Vitamins and minerals per serving (when baked and eaten with the skin): C (43% of the Daily Value), B_6 (35% DV), thiamin (15% DV), niacin (17% DV), riboflavin (4% DV), potassium (24% DV), manganese (23% DV), magnesium (14% DV), phosphorus (12% DV), iron (15% DV), zinc (4% DV), calcium (2% DV)
- Fiber per serving: 19% DV
- ORAC score: 313

Be aware that you lose vitamin C in cooking. And if you buy potato chips and French fries without the skins, they have fewer nutrients still—plus added fat and sodium.

ORANGES

Oranges at a Glance
- Pigments: beta-cryptoxanthin, zeaxanthin, lutein
- Other phytochemicals: hesperetin, limonin, nomilin, phytoene, phytofluene, d-limonene, beta-sitosterol, glutathione, D-glucaric acid
- Serving size: one orange
- Vitamins and minerals per serving: C (130% of the Daily Value), folate (12% DV), potassium (12% DV), thiamin (7% DV), niacin (4% DV), calcium (6% DV), magnesium (4% DV)
- Fiber per serving: 12% DV
- ORAC score: 750

There's a saying among Florida orange growers: "Ponce de León came looking for the Fountain of Youth. But in fact he brought it with him." This fountain of youth consisted of seeds for the orange tree.

If oranges really are an elixir of life, then part of their power clearly derives from their storehouse of vitamin C. This vitamin is one of the body's premier antioxidants. It also boosts immunity and helps the body absorb iron from food. An adequate supply in the diet prevents the disease scurvy, which used to kill sailors on long voyages. More than half of Vasco da Gama's crew died from scurvy on his first trip around the Cape of Good Hope in the late 1490s. Finally in the mid-1700s, the Scottish naval surgeon James Lind discovered a remedy: Dramatic cures were possible if the sailors simply ate oranges and lemons. The key, of course, was their vitamin C content.

Oranges are not only the master of the high C's. They also excel in other disease-banishing compounds, including limonoids and flavonoids.

QUICK 'N' EASY

Remember that salads aren't only about vegetables. Fruits add contrasting flavors and textures, which can perk up any dish. For example, mandarin orange slices right out of the can are delicious in a spinach salad. And you get an added bonus: The vitamin C in the oranges helps your body absorb the iron in the spinach.

For a classy dessert, add a splash of Grand Marnier to berries and orange slices. Grand Marnier is liqueur flavored with the dried peel of green oranges from the West Indian island of Curaçao.

Heart-Healthy Hesperetin

The main flavonoid in oranges is called *hesperetin*. It is also found in mandarins, lemons, limes, and, to a lesser extent, grapefruit—that is, citrus fruits that are high in vitamin C. Scientists suspect that this is no coincidence. Think of some inseparable couples from the movies—dance partners like Fred Astaire and Ginger Rogers or comedians like Laurel and Hardy. Each one needs the other to do his or her job properly. Vitamin C and hesperetin function like that in oranges. They are a team. According to antioxidant expert Lester Packer, flavonoids such as hesperetin work to regenerate vitamin C back to its active antioxidant form after the vitamin has quenched a free radical.

If that were the only job hesperetin performed, it would be incredibly valuable. But hesperetin does a lot more. It is a heart-protecting, cancer-fighting, infection-stomping compound that should be in everyone's diet. In one set of lab tests, researchers found that hesperetin slowed the replication of several viruses, including polio, herpes, and flu. Between hesperetin and vitamin C, you have two powerful reasons to eat oranges when you feel under the weather.

Even when you're feeling fit, oranges are an important part of a healthy diet. The Nurses' Health Study found that male and female nurses lowered their risks of stroke by 25 percent just by drinking a glass of orange juice a day. Other studies have shown that oranges promote heart health. Researchers in Italy have found that hesperetin reduces inflammation, lowers hypertension, increases "good" cholesterol, and lowers the "bad."

Are you wondering how hesperetin does all this? Elzbieta Kurowska at the University of Western Ontario wanted to know, too. Through a series of test-tube, animal, and human experiments, she has begun unraveling at least one of hesperetin's secrets. Kurowska found that hesperetin restricts the liver's production of compounds called cholesteryl esters that are major constituents of "bad" cholesterol, or LDL. Without them, the liver cannot make LDL. It's as if a bakery had orders for 20 angel food cakes, but was unable to whip them up because it had no egg whites.

Meet the Other Members of the Cardiac Team

Hesperetin is great, but it is just one of *five* heart-healthy substances in oranges. The next three are familiar friends:

- The soluble fiber pectin, which reduces cholesterol by scooping it up in the gut and escorting it out of the body, like a bouncer at a bar.
- Potassium, which helps lower blood pressure.
- Folate, which fights heart disease by ridding the body of excess homocysteine, a highly damaging compound that some scientists think contributes more to heart disease than cholesterol.

The last is an orange-yellow carotenoid called *beta-cryptoxanthin*. Its mechanism of action is not well understood, but there are some intriguing indications that it plays an important role in heart health. One study compared the residents of Belfast, Ireland, with the lucky people of Toulouse, France, who have four to eight times less heart disease. Researchers wanted to find out why, so they compared blood levels of the major antioxidant vitamins and carotenoids in the two populations. There were two striking differences. In the heart-healthy citizens of Toulouse, levels of beta-cryptoxanthin and another carotenoid called *lutein* were twice as high. The French participants got most of their cryptoxanthin from oranges. Their lutein came from broccoli and Brussels sprouts. It could just be that the key to the French paradox isn't red wine, after all, but fruits and vegetables!

QUICK 'N' EASY

Looking for something more exotic than a simple glass of OJ with breakfast? Here are two suggestions:

- Orange juice makes a great base for smoothies. Pour some into the blender along with strawberries, peaches, and a banana—or any other fruit you like. Raspberries, kiwi fruit, blackberries, and mango are all great, too. The banana gives the smoothie a creamy texture. For an even more "milk shakey" feel, peel the banana first and pop it in the freezer, so it's nice and cold. Nonfat yogurt can also enhance the smooth texture.
- For another tasty but simple drink, mix some juice in the blender along with—trust us—fresh spinach leaves. Does it sound outrageous? Try it once and we guarantee you'll be hooked. The resulting drink tastes a whole lot like orange juice, but less acidic. Your spinach-orange juice will come out a refreshing green color, with a pretty foam on top. Best of all, the vitamin C in the juice helps you absorb the iron in the spinach. It's great for women who need to boost their iron.

Eat to Beat Cancer

In a number of studies, oranges and other citrus fruits have also been shown to lower the risks of certain cancers, including stomach, mouth, and esophageal tumors. But why? Najla Guthrie at the University of Western Ontario decided to find out. She tested a number of the phytochemicals in oranges for their anti-cancer effects, and she began with hesperetin. Remarkably, she found it to be even more effective at slowing the proliferation of breast cancer cells than genistein—the highly touted cancer-fighting compound in soy. Still, hesperetin was far less effective than orange juice as a whole. Clearly hesperetin was not doing the job alone. Guthrie began to look beyond the flavonoids to another class of compounds called *limonoids,* part of the terpene family.

As it turns out, limonoids are found in the peel, membranes, seeds, and juice of the orange. These are not compounds you would want to eat plain. The two major limonoids in seeds— *limonin* and *nomilin*—are extremely bitter. But in the juice, these limonoids come bound to sugars, with health effects that are nothing but sweet. In test-tube experiments with breast cancer cells, Guthrie found that the limonoid compounds were up to 45 times more effective than hesperetin at blocking tumor formation! Other researchers have found that the limonoids inhibit lung, skin, and stomach cancers. The compounds appear to act in two ways—by stimulating the enzymes that detoxify carcinogens and by inducing abnormal cells to commit suicide.

As if that news isn't good enough, oranges also contain another terpene called *d-limonene,* which seems to help disarm a range of carcinogens, including one of the major nitrosamines in tobacco smoke. You can find limonene in orange juice, but there's even more in the peel, because it's one of those compounds that plants use to repel insects—and fruits obviously need most of that protection on the outside. (As an insect repellent, limonene appears to be effective. It's the active ingredient in Orange Guard, a household spray that gets rid of ants and cockroaches, yet can be used around food, pets, and children.)

In addition, the orange-yellow pigment beta-cryptoxanthin could also turn out to have cancer-fighting properties. Lab research in Japan has shown that cryptoxanthin's anti-cancer potential is five times greater than beta-carotene's in certain tests. In a series of broad population studies as well, high consumption of beta-cryptoxanthin has correlated with lower rates of breast and cervical cancer in women.

Boosting Limonene

Cancer-crushing limonene is the major component of orange-, lemon-, mandarin-, and grapefruit-peel oils. It is also found in juice, but the juice alone does not deliver enough limonene to achieve optimal health benefits. People of the Mediterranean region consume far more limonene than Americans do—frequently adding orange and lemon zest to breads, putting entire citrus slices into casseroles, and including candied peels in desserts. Is it mere coincidence that they also have lower cancer rates? Dr. Iman Hakim at the Arizona Cancer Center does not think so. She examined the eating habits of 475 Arizonans and discovered that those who used lemon or orange peels in cooking—as little as once a month—reduced their risks of squamous cell carcinoma of the skin by 50 percent.

Here are some suggestions for boosting limonene intake:

- Add orange and lemon zest or citrus slices to cooked dishes.
- Make Mediterranean-style lemonade by putting whole lemons into the blender. You will not only get limonene from the peel, but also extra limonin and nomilin from the seeds.
- Buy orange juice with pulp.
- Squeeze your own juice. Dr. Hakim has studied commercial juices and found that limonene levels vary dramatically depending on the packaging. "Limonene has a high affinity to fats and lipids, including wax," she says. "It can be absorbed by the packaging of waxed containers after two weeks on the shelf." To get the most limonene in a glass of juice, then, your best bet is to squeeze it fresh. The next best option is to buy juice in a can or glass bottle.

You Can't Judge an Orange by Its Peel

Florida's Valencia oranges do not generally look as perfect as California's navel oranges. That's partly a result of the Floridian climate. During summer thunderstorms, high winds can whip an orange tree's branches against the outside of the fruit, causing minor cuts known as windscars. Rest assured these blemishes do not affect the quality of the fruit inside, which is just as sweet and juicy as ever.

You may notice something else about the appearance of Valencias. These oranges sometimes have green in their peels when they're perfectly ripe. That's because they remain on the tree for 13 to 17 months before being picked. "They're still on the tree while a new crop is starting to grow," says Mohamed Ismail, scientific research director for the Florida Department of Citrus. When the trees flower in the spring and new fruits start to form, the trees produce extra chlorophyll, some of which is taken up by the more mature fruits. Again, this is not a drawback. "Oranges that have 'regreened' may actually be sweeter because they are extra ripe," says Ismail.

One shopping tip: If you're looking for oranges to juice, Florida's Valencia oranges are more suitable than California's navels because they come from a wetter environment. But that extra juice also means that Valencias develop a thinner skin, because the fruit inside expands and presses against the outside. That makes them harder to peel. California's navel oranges, by contrast, are regarded by many people as superior for eating, because they have a thicker skin that is relatively easy to peel off.

Tangerines

Tangerines always seem exotic, and with good reason. They're a type of mandarin orange, and mandarins originated in China. Despite the Asian connection, tangerines got their name because the first ones sent to Europe were shipped from Tangier, Morocco, in 1841.

If you like oranges, you'll love tangerines. They're easier to eat than oranges. In fact, they're known as "zipper fruits" because the thin skins peel off so easily. Once peeled, their sections also pull apart more easily than those of the orange. That means there's no excuse not to eat them! They're also loaded with protective phyto-chemicals—some of them different from the ones found in oranges. Take a look:

- Pigments: beta-cryptoxanthin, lutein
- Other phytochemicals: tangeretin, nobiletin, *d*-limonene
- Serving size: one tangerine
- Vitamins and minerals per serving: A (15% of the Daily Value), C (50% DV), folate (4% DV), potassium (4% DV)
- Fiber per serving: 8% DV
- ORAC score: not available

In addition to a powerful dose of vitamin C, tangerines contain a duo of health-promoting flavonoids, including one that was actually named for the fruit—*tangeretin*. The other one is called *nobiletin*. Scientists have observed that these flavonoids function as both anti-inflammatories and blood thinners, indicating that they may help prevent heart attacks, although this has not yet been demonstrated. These flavonoids also slow the growth of both skin and breast cancer cells in test-tube experiments. Researchers at the University of Western Ontario gave rats orange juice in place of drinking water and found that tangeretin was 36 times stronger than hesperetin at stopping the proliferation of these cancer cells. Nobiletin was almost as strong.

Another good choice: clementines, also called Algerian tangerines. Clementines were first grown in Algeria in the early 20th century by Father Clément Rodier, who accidentally created the hybrid. Buy these fruits by the crate around Christmastime and leave those darling clementines out on the table for hungry friends and relatives. They're virtually free of seeds and also peel in a snap. Amid all the tempting holiday treats, they'll still find an eager following.

GRAPEFRUIT

Grapefruit at a Glance
- Pigments: lycopene and beta-carotene (pink grapefruit only)
- Other phytochemicals: naringenin, D-glucaric acid, *d*-limonene, ferulic acid, hesperetin, quercetin, kaempferol, limonin, nomilin, beta-sitosterol, glutathione
- Serving size: one half grapefruit
- Vitamins and minerals per serving: A (12 to 50% of the Daily Value, for pink grapefruit only), C (70% DV), potassium (5% DV), thiamin (3% DV), folate (3% DV), magnesium (3% DV)
- Fiber per serving: 6% DV
- ORAC score (for pink grapefruit): 483

Two years ago, China opened its markets to an exotic new fruit from the United States. Known to botanists by the alluring name *Citrus paradisi*, it's better known to Americans as plain, simple grapefruit—a name it acquired because it grows in bunches like grapes. But "citrus of paradise" might be a more appropriate appellation, given the health benefits. As the first Ocean Spray Ruby Reds went on sale in China, the *New York Times* reported that some people drove as much as two hours to market to purchase them. Who could resist such a sales pitch?—"Grapefruits from Florida . . . Famous Brand Name . . . Healthy and Tasty . . . Good for Your Blood and for Beauty."

We should all be as excited about grapefruit. It's a top health-promoting food.

A Phytochemical Cocktail with an Anti-cancer Punch

As a member of the citrus family, grapefruit naturally excels in vitamin C. A single serving (half a grapefruit) delivers 70 percent of your daily quota. And being high in C, it also contains a storehouse of antioxidant-regenerating flavonoids.

The main flavonoid in grapefruit is called *naringenin,* and it's yet another cancer fighter. A number of lab studies show that it's not as strong as quercetin, but that's no reason to omit it from the diet. When epidemiologist Loïc Le Marchand of the University of Hawaii compared the diets of 582 lung-cancer patients and an equal number of cancer-free controls, he found that three foods stood out for their apparent ability to reduce lung-cancer risk, in addition to carotenoid-rich fruits and vegetables. These three were apples and onions (with their quercetin) and white grapefruit (with its naringenin). According to Le Marchand, naringenin guards against cancer by reducing the activity of the phase 1 enzymes, which can create carcinogens out of harmless substances.

In addition to naringenin and other flavonoids, grapefruit serves up a whole phytochemical cocktail, including cancer-crushing limonene, limonin, and nomilin. The red and pink varieties of grapefruit ratchet up their tumor-fighting ability still further with lycopene. And on top of all this you get ferulic acid, which inhibits the activation of a carcinogen in tobacco called NNK. "Ferulic acid is only moderately inhibitory of cancer," says Robert Teel, professor of physiology and pharmacology at Loma Linda University. "But when you eat fruits and vegetables, you get a mixture of these compounds. It may very well be that the interaction is more beneficial than the compounds by themselves." In other words, the health-promoting activity of an entire grapefruit is greater than the sum of its parts.

Heart Check

Have you noticed the little red hearts with white check marks inside them on certain packaged foods? They're the American Heart Association's sign of a heart-healthy item. Grapefruit juice more than qualifies, thanks to its low fat and high vitamin C. In addition, the juice also boasts potassium and folate, and it's a great source of cholesterol-lowering pectin. And that's not all. Grapefruit is also one of the best sources of D-*glucaric acid*, yet another cholesterol-lowering compound.

If there were a check mark for cancer-fighting foods, grapefruit juice would qualify for that, too. In addition to lowering cholesterol, D-glucaric acid detoxifies a number of carcinogens, including various nitrosamines and heterocyclic amines. In one recent study, Zbigniew Walaszek of the AMC Cancer Research Center in Denver found that when he exposed rats to a carcinogen, they developed 60 percent less colon cancer if he also added a derivative of D-glucaric acid to their diets. He has also had good results inhibiting skin, lung, and mammary cancers in rodents. Walaszek is now beginning very early trials in people, both smokers and non-smokers, to see if short-term doses can affect cancer-causing genes called oncogenes.

DON'T MISS OUT ON GLUCARIC ACID

Just as quickly as natural cancer-fighting substances are discovered, supplement manufacturers race to bottle them. The problem with this approach is that foods are complex mixtures of hundreds of chemicals. If you single out one, you neglect other good stuff. D-glucaric acid is one compound that you can easily miss out on unless you eat your grapefruit, apples, and broccoli.

Food	D-Glucaric Acid
Grapefruit	360*
Alfalfa sprouts	350

Food	D-Glucaric Acid
McIntosh apples	350
Broccoli	340
Granny Smith apples	340
Brussels sprouts	270
Tomatoes	210
Cauliflower	180
Cherries	140
Apricots	140
Oranges	130
Spinach	110

*measured in milligrams per 100 grams (about 3.5 ounces) of food
Source: Zbigniew Walaszek, AMC Cancer Research Center

Important!

As healthy as grapefruit juice is, it should not be consumed with certain prescription drugs, including many of the calcium-channel blockers that treat hypertension and a number of the statin drugs that are used to lower cholesterol. That's because naringenin and other compounds in grapefruit juice deactivate enzymes that normally degrade much of the drug before it enters into your bloodstream. With less of the enzyme in action, more of the drug gets into your system and may deliver an overdose. (Unfortunately, the additional amount is highly unpredictable, so you can't compensate by simply lowering your prescription.)

Dr. Garvan Kane at the Mayo Clinic recently reviewed the medical literature and concluded that a number of other drugs may interact with grapefruit juice, too. If you're a grapefruit juice drinker, be sure to ask your physician or your pharmacist about possible interactions with any new prescriptions.

Lemons

Lemons contain many of the excellent phytonutrients that you find in other citrus fruits, and they are rich in vitamin C. The only problem is, lemons are too sour for snacking. But here's a health-

QUICK 'N' EASY

If you still need help boosting your fruit intake, try joining a fruit-of-the-month club. The prices may be steeper than at your local market, but you can't beat the convenience and quality. Companies like Harry and David in Medford, Oregon (www.harrydavid.com), provide delicious selections year round, ranging from Royal Riviera pears to red bananas and honeybell tangelos. If it's citrus you love, check out Hale Indian River Groves in Wabasso, Florida (www.hales.com). They provide other fruits, too, but their citrus excels.

Enter "fruit of the month," "gift fruit," or "gift vegetables" into your Internet search engine to find still other sources of produce. Some examples:

- www.starorganic.com
- www.urbanorganic.com (for organic products shipped nationwide)
- www.deliciousorchardsnj.com

ful tip: Try squeezing lemon juice over vegetables and seafood instead of salt. The reduced salt intake helps prevent hypertension, and the cancer-fighting phytochemicals in lemons can only work to your benefit.

MANGOES

Mangoes at a Glance

- Pigments: beta-carotene, beta-cryptoxanthin, anthocyanins (one form of peonidin)
- Other phytochemicals: gallic acid, gallotannins, mangiferine, quercetin, kaempferol, syringic acid, phytoene, phytofluene
- Serving size: one mango
- Vitamins and minerals per serving: A (160% of the Daily Value), C (95% DV), B_6 (14% DV), E (10% DV), folate (7% DV), potassium (9% DV)

- Fiber per serving: 15% DV
- ORAC score: 302 (measured by Brunswick Labs)

As Buddhist missionaries fanned out across Asia thousands of years ago, they took with them the seed of one of their favorite fruits, the mango. Not only was it one of the most succulent fruits imaginable, but it also had symbolic importance. Legend has it that Buddha, tired and weary one day, was presented with a grove of mango trees in which to rest. Ever since then, the mango tree has been associated with wishes that are granted. In Indian villages, mango leaves are used as decorations at weddings to ensure that the newlyweds will have many children. And when a son is born, villagers announce the happy event by adorning their doorways with mango leaves. In fact, leaves of the mango tree are used at almost every festival and religious celebration in India to ensure good luck.

As far as we're concerned, mangoes themselves are a wish come true. Savoring a juicy ripe mango is about as close to nirvana as you can get in this life. The taste is exquisite—at once sweet, complex, and assertive, with overtones of citrus and jasmine. That's why mangoes go just as well in spicy salsas and chutneys as they do in desserts. Pair mango with ginger, chilies, and cilantro, and you can make a great accompaniment for trout or salmon. In Brazil, you can even find mango sushi. "It sounds strange at first, but mangoes go well with soy sauce," says Richard Campbell, curator of tropical fruit at Fairchild Tropical Garden in Coral Gables, Florida. "They are sophisticated fruits with a whole suite of aromatic flavor components that you don't find in fruits from temperate climates."

There has been little research on mangoes, but they are clearly a healthy food. In one study, researchers in New Zealand attempted to figure out why the native Maori people have lower cancer rates than New Zealanders of European descent. The researchers singled out 25 foods that the Maoris eat in far greater quantities and then tested these foods in the laboratory. Six of them—including watercress, papaya, taro leaves, green banana, and mango—showed potent anti-cancer effects. Just why was not clear, but the researchers suspected that the cancer-squelching components in these protective foods might include carotenoids and flavonoids.

> **Mango Trivia**
>
> Did you know that the irregular shape of the mango inspired the paisley pattern? The paisley design originated in northern India, where the local mangoes have the classic S-shape twist to them. Local artisans embroidered these skewed patterns into elaborate Kashmiri shawls, which British merchants carried back with them from India. Scottish weavers then took up the design. It became known for the town that produced the most of this patterned fabric—Paisley, near Glasgow in southern Scotland.

Mangoes do contain a nice amount of beta-carotene, plus beta-cryptoxanthin, phytoene, and phytofluene. They also pack cancer-fighting quercetin. Roll these together with the antioxidant vitamin C, and you have a winner. All these phytochemicals fight cancer. But there's more. "There's a class of phenolic acids in tropical fruits that you don't find in the standard fruits and vegetables, like carrots or potatoes," says food chemist Stephen Talcott of the University of Florida in Gainesville. "Slice mangoes open and they don't brown, the way an apple or banana does." The primary phenolic acid Talcott has isolated in mangoes is gallic acid, a potent antioxidant that's also found in grapes. He suspects that gallic acid and related compounds may account for the anti-cancer effect that his colleague Susan S. Percival has seen from mango extracts in the lab.

In one preliminary trial, Percival put mouse cells in petri dishes along with all the nutrients they would need to grow. She then added a cancer-causing chemical. Normal cells stop growing when they start touching other cells around them, so that they form a clean, single layer of cells in the dish. Cancer cells, however, keep right on growing, heaping up into little piles of cells called foci. When Percival added carcinogens to the petri dishes, lots of foci formed among the mouse cells; when Percival added mango extracts to the mix, the number of foci was dramatically reduced. Percival took the experiment one step further and divided the mango extracts into two fractions, or parts—the fat-soluble compounds (including carotenoids) and the water-soluble compounds (including phenolics). "When I did the calculations, I found the water-soluble fraction was ten times more effective than the carotenoid fraction," says Percival. "We're very interested in finding out what is in that water-soluble fraction."

How to Skin a Mango

Exotic fruits can be puzzling, with their unfamiliar looks. How can you tell when they're ripe? Luckily, picking a great mango is not really that mysterious. The surest sign of a scrumptious fruit is a deliciously flowery fragrance. A ripe mango should also be soft enough to yield to a slight squeeze. (Skin color is not the best guide, as different varieties of mangoes have different hues—some orange-red at maturity, others yellow when fully ripe.) Do make sure that the skin is not shriveled, as this indicates an overripe fruit.

The trickiest part of preparing mangoes is slicing them up. But with a little practice, it's not that difficult, says Richard Campbell, curator of tropical fruit at Fairchild Tropical Garden. He should know. Campbell and his assistants slice up two to three tons of mangoes a year for Fairchild's annual mango festival in July. "There are many ways to skin a mango," he reports. But this is the simplest.

Hold the mango in your hand so that it lies flat in your palm. With a sharp knife, slice the skin in thin strips off the top half. Cut off all of the fruit above the large, flat seed. Then flip the fruit over and repeat the process on the other side. Pare away any fruit that is still left clinging to the seed. Don't try this on a cutting board, warns Campbell, because the fruit is too slippery. "You have to hold it in your hand," he says.

Another method that is very popular in India for snacking is to take the whole mango and knead it between your fingers or roll it

QUICK 'N' EASY
Mango smoothies couldn't be easier to make. Just peel and remove the pit from some mangoes—or buy bags of frozen mango chunks—and toss them into the blender along with vanilla yogurt and orange juice or soy milk. That's all you need for a refreshing summer drink.

on the table to soften up the pulp inside. When it feels mushy, slice off the top and suck the mango out—juice, pulp, and all.

CANTALOUPE

The Bible tells us that when the Israelites left Egypt to wander in the wilderness with Moses for 40 years, they lamented leaving behind many of their favorite foods, including melons. Was the melon of their dreams the cantaloupe? This fruit is of Persian origin, but it is supposed to have been found in the Mediterranean by 2400 B.C.— and its absence would certainly be worth mourning. Of all the melons, it is the most nutritious, thanks largely to its beta-carotene and vitamin C, a potent combination for fighting both heart disease and cancer. The cantaloupe also contains a hefty dose of potassium, which helps regulate blood pressure. Take a look:

- Pigments: beta-carotene, alpha-carotene
- Other phytochemicals: rutin, ferulic acid, glutathione
- Serving size: one cup, chopped
- Vitamins and minerals per serving: A (103% of the Daily Value), C (113% DV), folate (7% DV), potassium (14% DV), magnesium (5% DV), iron (2% DV), calcium (2% DV)
- Fiber per serving: 5% DV
- ORAC score: 252

Of course, picking out a juicy, ripe cantaloupe can seem like a challenge. You see people in markets thumping and shaking melons in an attempt to find a good one. But the surest way to pick a winner is to sniff the end for a sweet fragrance. If the fruit doesn't smell sweet and inviting, don't buy it; cantaloupe does not ripen further after it leaves the vine. Also, look for a raised "netting" covering the entire rind—which, incidentally, should be beige rather than a dull green.

Melon trivia: The fruit we call the cantaloupe is actually a muskmelon. The true cantaloupe—named for Cantalupo, Italy— has a warty, gourdlike exterior. It is rarely grown outside the Mediterranean region.

PUMPKINS

Pumpkins at a Glance

- Pigments: alpha-carotene, beta-carotene, lutein, zeaxanthin
- Other phytochemicals: ferulic acid, glutamic acid, lignans
- Serving size: one-half cup, cooked
- Vitamins and minerals per serving: A (27% of the Daily Value), C (10% DV), E (8% DV), folate (3% DV), potassium (8% DV), iron (4% DV)
- Fiber per serving: 6% DV
- ORAC score: 404 (measured by Brunswick Labs)

Long before Columbus landed in the New World, Native Americans were cultivating pumpkins. They grew them together with corn and beans in a clever style called the "three sisters." First they would build up mounds of earth and plant a grain of corn—the first sister—in the middle of each one. Next to the corn they planted beans—the second sister. As the beans grew, their tendrils would twist around the cornstalks. This helped both plants by eliminating the need for bean poles and strengthening the cornstalks, too. The last sister in the trio was the pumpkin, planted between the mounds. The pumpkin leaves shaded the ground, keeping the moisture level up and the weeds down.

When the crop was ready for harvest, Native Americans knew many uses for the pumpkin. Although their word for pumpkins and other squash was *askutasquash* ("something eaten raw"), they probably did not eat this tough winter squash straight. Instead we know they roasted pumpkin strips over the fire and dried pumpkin strips to take on hunting expeditions. They also roasted the seeds for both food and medicines.

When the Pilgrims arrived in Massachusetts in 1620, it didn't take them long to realize that pumpkins were one of the staples that they could rely on. Early records indicate that the settlers ate pumpkins at their second Thanksgiving celebration. They didn't have pie as we know it today, but they made a sweet dessert by filling the inside of a pumpkin with milk, spices, and honey. Baked in hot ashes, the pumpkin turned into a delicious concoction. The settlers also made pumpkin soup and even pumpkin beer. An old American folk song, written perhaps as early as 1643, told how important this humble fruit was to the survival of our first immigrants:

If flesh meat be wanting to fill up our dish,
We have carrots and pumpkins and turnips and fish. . . .
We have pumpkin at morning and pumpkin at noon
If it were not for pumpkins, we would be undone.

The pumpkin continued to be part of American life for centuries afterward, right down to this bizarre footnote: When Whittaker Chambers accused Alger Hiss of being a Communist Party member in 1948 (setting off the wave of hysteria that came to be known as McCarthyism), Chambers brought federal investigators to his Maryland farm to show them incriminating documents he claimed Hiss had given him. Chambers dramatically produced the microfilmed papers—not from his desk, but from a hollowed out pumpkin in his pumpkin patch, where he had stashed them for safekeeping. They became known as the "pumpkin papers."

Alpha Comes Before Beta—Maybe

Today, pumpkins have largely been relegated to jack-o'-lanterns and Thanksgiving pies. That's too bad, because they contain a treasure trove of beneficial carotenoids. After sweet potatoes and carrots, pumpkins boast more beta-carotene than any other food in our diets. As if this weren't bounty enough, they are also the richest dietary source of cancer-fighting alpha-carotene, and they contain smaller amounts of lutein and zeaxanthin, too. That's a great combo. Loïc Le Marchand of the University of Hawaii assessed the food preferences of 332 men and women with lung cancer, then compared them with the diets of 865 cancer-free controls. Overall, the healthy controls ate the most alpha-carotene, beta-carotene, and lutein. You can get all three in pumpkins.

Although alpha-carotene is less well known than beta-carotene, it could turn out to be an even better cancer fighter. In a series of studies, Michiaki Murakoshi of the Kyoto Prefectural University of Medicine in Japan coated human cancer cells in the lab with carotenoids. Alpha-carotene was ten times more effective at reducing their proliferation than beta-carotene. Murakoshi also found that alpha-carotene outperformed beta-carotene at squelching skin, liver, and lung tumors in mice. It slashed the number of lung tumors by 70 percent. Much work still needs to be done. But increasingly, studies suggest that a combination of all the major carotenoids offers the best protection.

THE BEST SOURCES OF ALPHA- AND BETA-CAROTENE

Beta-carotene is one of the most common carotenoids in the diet. But certain bright orange foods, like carrots and pumpkins, also contain substantial amounts of alpha-carotene. Here are the top dietary sources for both.

Food	Beta-Carotene	Alpha-Carotene
Sweet potato, baked	9.5*	0*
Carrots, raw	8.8	4.6
Pumpkin, canned	6.9	4.8
Kale, cooked	6.2	0
Spinach, raw	5.6	0
Butternut squash	4.6	1.1
Collard greens, cooked	4.4	0.1

*measured in milligrams per 100 grams (about 3.5 ounces) of food
Source: VERIS Research Information Service

Eat the Seeds, Too!

Come Halloween, we carve pumpkins into jack-o'-lanterns. But what happens to the seeds that we scoop out? Don't throw them away. The seeds have a delightful, nutty taste and make a nice addition to salads, soups, and casseroles. They're also a delicious peanuty snack all by themselves.

Best of all, they're healthy, too. In Germany, Turkey, and Bulgaria, pumpkin seeds have been used as a traditional remedy for benign enlargement of the prostate gland—a problem that plagues half of all men over age 50. In one randomized, double-blind study of 53 men in Sweden and Denmark, those who took a combination of pumpkin seeds and saw palmetto showed significant relief of symptoms. The researchers did not know why, but speculated that it's because the seeds are rich in beta-sitosterol, which has been shown in animal tests to slow abnormal cell proliferation (and to lower cholesterol, too!). Botanist James A. Duke, author of *The Green Pharmacy,* adds that pumpkin seeds also contain beneficial compounds called *cucurbitacins.* These compounds reduce the conversion of the male sex hormone testosterone into a related hormone, dihydrotestosterone, which stimulates the proliferation of prostate cells. Although there is far more research on saw palmetto, the evidence for pumpkin seeds is strong enough that Duke himself takes a daily mixture of fresh pumpkin seeds, saw palmetto, and selenium-rich Brazil nuts, since epidemiological studies have correlated a high selenium intake with low rates of prostate cancer. In addition, he eats plenty of lycopene-rich tomato products.

Pumpkin seeds are also rich in protein and minerals such as iron, magnesium, manganese, phosphorus, and zinc. And, an ounce of seeds contains 1.1 grams of fiber. Although pumpkin seeds are relatively high in fat, their oils are mainly the healthful monounsaturated and polyunsaturated kinds.

To roast the seeds from your pumpkin, start by rinsing them in a colander. Then, pull off the strings, and pat the seeds dry between towels. When the seeds are thoroughly cleaned, toss them in a bowl with a little olive oil. Spread evenly on a baking sheet, lightly salt, and bake at 375°F for 45 minutes, turning occasionally.

From Jack-be-Little to Mammoth Gold

Pumpkins come in many varieties, with such evocative names as Spooktacular, Funny Face, Jumpin' Jack, Munchkin, and Sweetie Pie. They also run the gamut in sizes, from Jack-be-Little miniatures to giant Mammoth Golds that weigh in at hundreds of pounds. The current world record holder topped the scales at 1,131 pounds!

If you want to cook with fresh pumpkins, look for ones that are labeled as "pie pumpkins" or "sweet pumpkins." These are smaller than typical jack-o'-lantern pumpkins, and their flesh is sweeter, less stringy, and less watery. They go nicely in recipes for everything from soup to whole wheat pumpkin bread. Don't be afraid to experiment. Your only limit is the extent of your imagination. As one teacher points out, "Cinderella's pumpkin was used as a coach."

SQUASH

There are more than 40 different types of squash, ranging from summer's yellow crookneck to the rich winter varieties—acorn, buttercup, Hubbard, and many more. It is impossible to list all the phytochemicals in a group that is so diverse. But one rule of thumb will not fail you: The darker the squash, the more nutrients it contains. That means that the winter squashes in general, with their rich orange flesh, are better sources of carotenoids—not to mention vitamins, minerals, and fiber—than the pallid summer squashes.

Even the most colorful of the summer varieties, zucchini, is basically white on the inside—and at 95 percent water, it contains only modest levels of nutrients. Definitely wash your zucchini, but don't peel it, because most of the nutrients are in the skin.

Here's a quick comparison of vitamins, minerals, and fiber in a composite of winter versus summer squashes.

Summer Squash:
- Serving size: one-half cup
- Vitamins and minerals per serving: A (5% of the Daily Value), C (8% DV), folate (5% DV), manganese (10% DV), potassium (5% DV)
- Fiber per serving: 5% DV

Winter Squash:
- Serving size: one-half cup
- Vitamins and minerals per serving: A (73% of the Daily Value), C (17% DV), folate (7% DV), manganese (11% DV), potassium (13% DV)
- Fiber per serving: 12% DV

Bear in mind that these are averages. Precise composition will differ with the variety of squash. For example, butternut squash delivers a whopping 143 percent of your daily vitamin A needs rather than the 73 percent in the composite.

APRICOTS

Apricots at a Glance
- Pigments: beta-carotene, lycopene
- Other phytochemicals: chlorogenic acid, geraniol, quercetin, D-glucaric acid
- Serving size: 3 apricots
- Vitamins and minerals per serving: A (55% of the Daily Value), C (20% DV), potassium (9% DV), iron (3% DV), magnesium (2% DV), calcium (2% DV)
- Fiber per serving: 12% DV
- ORAC score: 164

In the early part of the 20th century, the Hunza River Valley of central Asia proved a magnet for explorers and adventure seekers, who were drawn to some of the most far-flung outposts of the British Empire. The Hunza River Valley was a place of breathtaking mountains and dramatic, rugged scenery in what is today part of northern Pakistan. But in addition to the dramatic landscape, something else impressed Western travelers—the robust health of the Hunzukut people. They appeared to live well into old age, free of heart disease and cancer. In part, this was no doubt because they got plenty of exercise, breathed pure air, and drank unpolluted glacier water. But clearly, their diet of fresh fruits, vegetables, and whole grains also played a role. In particular, visitors noticed that the Hunzukuts ate astonishing quantities of apricots. As one visitor described the local four-meal-a-day diet, it consisted of flatbread with fresh or boiled apricots for breakfast; dried apricots, boiled vegetables, and flatbread for lunch; apricot soup for dinner; and vegetables and fruit for late-evening supper. The Hunzukut men joked that their wives would not live any place where apricots did not grow. Maybe the next time we're all in the market for real estate, we should try telling the agent that we need apricot trees!

> ## QUICK 'N' EASY
>
> Although apricots are delicious fresh, they are generally eaten dried. Stash a box in your desk drawer for mid-afternoon munchies. Some of the best dried apricots come from Turkey, where a tempting dessert called *kaysi dolma* is made from dried apricots, sweet cream, and walnuts.

CORN

Corn at a Glance

- Pigments: lutein, zeaxanthin
- Other phytochemicals: eugenol, ferulic acid, isoquercitrin
- Serving size: one-half cup
- Vitamins and minerals per serving: C (8% of the Daily Value), thiamin (13% DV), folate (10% DV), niacin (7% DV), phosphorus (8% DV), potassium (3% DV), zinc (3% DV)
- Fiber per serving: 12% DV
- ORAC: 402

In the Midwest, they have a special name for corn. They call it Prairie Gold. Americans have devised a myriad of uses for this versatile grain. We eat it straight, feed it to livestock, press it for oil, mill it for starch, convert it to corn syrup, and derive more products from it than you could ever imagine—ethanol fuel, printer's ink, "packing peanuts," disposable diapers, noncorrosive road de-icer, and a whole host of biodegradable plastics that are gentler on the environment than petroleum-based products. From corncob pipes to cornbread, corn is an ingrained part of our culture, with sometimes surprising results. Dozens of towns across the Midwest have drawn late-summer visitors to their "maize mazes," all built from carefully planted corn rows. Even quirkier, Mitchell, South Dakota, boasts the Mitchell Corn Palace, with its eclectic mix of onion domes and minarets, not to mention murals that are fashioned every year from corn and grasses. What other food inspires stunts that are as corny as Kansas in August?

Despite these zany sights, we can't deny a basic truth. In this country, "corn-fed" is a synonym for "wholesome." There's a reason for that.

A Cornucopia of Benefits

An average ear of sweet corn has 800 kernels, each of them a mini storehouse of carbohydrates, protein, vitamins, minerals, and fiber. Corn is a terrific source of thiamin, one of the B vitamins, which helps maintain the nervous system. It's also got plenty of niacin, which helps regulate cholesterol in the blood, and it's a source of folate, phosphorus, and fiber. Corn also has more protein than many vegetables. No wonder maize has sustained entire populations in Central and South America. (You may have heard that people in these regions pound the corn with lime, or calcium carbonate, to make the niacin more bioavailable. That is necessary with field corn, which is used for chips and tortillas, but in the sweet corn that we eat on the cob, niacin is readily available.)

Anyone who is interested only in vitamins and minerals, however, is overlooking another of corn's virtues that is right there in plain sight—the yellow pigments that give corn its golden hue. These pigments are called lutein and zeaxanthin.

Lutein and zeaxanthin are both members of the carotenoid family. Like other carotenoids, they also appear to help fight heart disease and cancer. But they play at least one role that is distinct from all the rest. Acting as antioxidants, they protect a supersensitive area of the eye called the macula. Without the macula, we would not have the sharp central vision that enables us to read fine print, drive a car, or make out the features of the person standing right in front of us. It is precisely this crucial part of vision that is lost in a devastating disease called age-related macular degeneration. This condition is the leading cause of blindness in the elderly. Lutein and zeaxanthin can help prevent it. But you won't get any in white corn, only yellow (or better yet, in very dark green vegetables, which contain even denser levels of these carotenoids).

Why Does Popcorn Pop?

Not just any corn will pop. It takes a special corn, with precisely the right amount of moisture on the inside, a thick hull on the outside, and a certain balance of starch granules. All three are crucial, says popcorn breeder Ken Ziegler of Iowa State University.

As a popcorn kernel heats up, the water inside turns to steam and presses outward. Unable to break through the strong hull, the steam pushes instead into the densely packed starch granules inside the kernel. Eventually the pressure becomes too great for even a strong hull to contain. The kernel explodes as the hull gives way. In the process, the escaping steam puffs up the starch granules, and the kernel turns itself inside out.

Because popped corn is mostly air by volume, it is a low-calorie snack, but it still delivers a small amount of protein and B vitamins. To jazz up popcorn without adding fat, the Popcorn Board recommends any of the following low-cal toppings: curry powder; dry Italian salad dressing mix; vegetable flakes; dried soup mix; dill weed; or powdered orange rind.

BANANAS

Bananas at a Glance
- Pigments: beta-carotene, alpha-carotene
- Other phytochemicals: kaempferol, quercetin, rutin, vanillic acid, fructooligosaccharides
- Serving size: one banana
- Vitamins and minerals per serving: A (9% of the Daily Value), C (15% DV), B_6 (33% DV), folate (6% DV), potassium (13% DV), magnesium (8% DV)
- Fiber per serving: 11% DV
- ORAC score: 221

Bananas were officially introduced into the United States at the celebration of the nation's first centennial in 1876. Just imagine the sight at the Philadelphia Centennial Exhibition, where bananas were wrapped in foil and sold as a great delicacy for 10 cents apiece! Bananas may have been new to Pennsylvanians in the 1800s, but they are perhaps the world's oldest cultivated fruit. They are believed to have originated in the jungles of Malaysia thousands of years ago. Before the birth of Christ, they were brought to India, where they became known as the "fruit of the wise men." According to Indian legend, sages meditated under the shady, green leaves of banana groves.

Like corn, the banana is a staple that has sustained populations. Also like corn, it has an astonishing array of uses, particularly in Africa and Asia, where almost every part of the plant is used for something. Food is only the most obvious. People use banana leaves for umbrellas, thatching, tablecloths, and disposable "plates." They pound the peels into poultices to treat wounds, thanks to the natural antiseptics in the inner peel. They use the ash to manufacture soap, and they process the sap into a dye. Where bananas grow wild, even their large, black seeds are harvested for decorative beads.

As Good as Medicine

As a food, bananas are a dense source of carbohydrates and also provide a hefty dose of potassium, which is a very good thing. Potassium is best known as a blood pressure regulator. That's because it reduces the formation of a chemical called angiotensin, which constricts blood vessels. Potassium also acts as a natural diuretic, causing the body to excrete both water and sodium. In fact, many cardiologists believe that high blood pressure is caused as much by low potassium as by high sodium.

Unfortunately, modern processed foods have stripped much of the potassium out of our diets, and at the same time they've added a mother lode of salt. Two hundred years ago, the average person consumed eight times more potassium than sodium. Today, the ratio is one to four in the opposite direction. No wonder hypertension is practically a national epidemic, afflicting half of all Americans in their 60s and two-thirds of those over 70.

Fortunately, eating potassium-rich foods like bananas often prevents or reduces high blood pressure. "High blood pressure is not an inherent part of aging," says Eva Obarzanek, a research nutritionist at the National Heart, Lung, and Blood Institute. Obarzanek helped conduct a now-famous study called Dietary Approaches to Stop Hypertension (DASH). In this study, 459 volunteers followed one of three diets for eight weeks. Those who achieved the best results were the participants on the so-called

DASH diet—a low-fat regimen with 10 daily servings of fruits and vegetables; two servings of low-fat dairy products; and two or less of fish, poultry, or lean meat. By following this diet, volunteers with high blood pressure reduced their systolic and diastolic blood pressure by 11.4 and 5.5 points, respectively—*without reducing their salt intake.* "That's comparable to what you achieve with medications," says Obarzanek. A large part of the reason was that participants were skipping high-fat foods and dining instead on potassium-rich foods like bananas and oranges.

Love, Money, and Potassium

Not only does a high-potassium diet reduce hypertension, but it also appears to reduce plaque formation in arteries, according to lab studies by David B. Young, a cardiovascular physiologist at the University of Mississippi Medical Center in Jackson and author of *The Role of Potassium in Preventive Cardiovascular Medicine.* The precise mechanism is not clear. But potassium is known to affect the internal signaling process within cells. Somehow, the cells produce fewer free radicals as a result—and a reduction in free radicals means less oxidation of LDL, or "bad" cholesterol. It is oxidation of LDL that sets in motion the chain of events leading to atherosclerosis and heart disease.

That's not all potassium does for you. It also turns down the activity of platelets, which cause the blood to clot. Of course you want blood to form a scab if you cut yourself. But blood can also clot with much less provocation. These unwanted clots account for about 80 percent of strokes. "Clinical studies show that there's a reduction in strokes on a high-potassium diet," says Young. "Potassium is one of those things like love and money that you just can't get too much of."

A Boon for Bones?

Everyone knows that calcium and vitamin D are essential for bone strength. But new research indicates that other minerals could play a supporting role, too, including two minerals that bananas have in abundance—potassium and magnesium. Katherine Tucker of Tufts University assessed the diets of 907 people, then took four measurements of bone strength for each participant. Those who ate the most fruits and vegetables in general—and foods rich in magnesium and potassium in particular—showed greater bone density than those who ate the least of these foods. Bananas were one of the top sources of both minerals in the foods the study participants ate. (Potassium is found in many other fruits and vegetables, too, including oranges, broccoli, and cantaloupe. Sources of magnesium include dark bread, orange juice, fish, spinach, chicken, peanut butter, and nuts.)

Nutritionist Susan New of the University of Surrey in England found very similar results when she studied 62 women aged 45 to 55. Those who ate fruits and vegetables rich in magnesium and potassium had greater bone density. Again, we would encourage you to consume the whole foods rather than mineral supplements, because the benefits could come from unidentified substances in these foods—or even a combination of factors.

Beneficial Bacteria

Bananas can aid the body in yet another way that most of us rarely think about—promoting colon health. That's because they contain an unusual type of fiber called—brace yourself—*short-chain fructooligosaccharides,* or FOS for short. These FOS are your colon's friend. They ferment in the gut, providing food for the beneficial bacteria that keep disease-causing microbes in check. These good bacteria even appear to protect against colon cancer, so it's a good idea to keep them happy and healthy. FOS can also benefit your bones indirectly. That's because they increase the acidity level in the colon, and greater acidity aids calcium absorption.

Plantains

Plantains resemble bananas, but bite into one, and you'll immediately know the difference. Whereas bananas store their carbohydrates in the form of sugar, plantains are more starchy. They are generally eaten boiled, steamed, baked, or fried and hence are known as "cooking bananas." They are a staple crop through much of Africa. In 1874, after spending 16 years in West Africa, the American missionary Robert Nassau wrote: "Even after the long interval to the present time, and tasting every variety of vegetable, I know none that I enjoy more than boiled ripe plantains."

Plantains are even richer in vitamins and minerals than bananas. A cup of plantains contains the following vitamins and minerals: A (28% of the Daily Value), C (28% DV), B_6 (19% DV), folate (10% DV), and potassium (20% DV), plus 20% of the daily requirement of fiber.

FROM THE SPICE CHEST: TURMERIC

As any self-respecting *Seinfeld* fan knows, there is a soup chef in New York City named Al Yeganeh—better known as the Soup Nazi, for his tendency to scold customers and even refuse to serve those who don't follow his rigid rules for ordering. Although the Soup Nazi became famous through a sitcom, he is a real person, and his little soup restaurant routinely draws lines that stretch to the end of the block. Our co-author Anne Underwood can testify to this, as Yeganeh's Soup Kitchen International is just two blocks from her office. (Once, the Soup Nazi even refused to give her bread because she didn't step immediately to the left after ordering.) All of this is a long way of saying that one of Yeganeh's finest soups—and the object of Kramer's desires in that *Seinfeld* episode—is a delightful Indian soup called mulligatawny. Mulligatawny is a delicious blend of lentils, nuts, carrots, onions, and spices. But it wouldn't be half the soup it is without a special ingredient: the yellow spice turmeric.

Turmeric is not only an essential ingredient of mulligatawny, but also the *sine qua non* of curry. Without turmeric in the mix, curry sauces would not have their characteristic golden hue. Without turmeric, curries would also be less healthy. Long before the development of refrigeration or even ice houses, people used turmeric to prevent meats from turning rancid, because the spice functions as a powerful antioxidant. Turmeric also works as a strong anti-inflammatory. That's an unbeatable combination. For centuries, the peoples of India have used turmeric in traditional Ayurvedic remedies to improve digestion, treat heart disease, and heal wounds. Scientific testing is starting to validate all of these uses. But the bulk of the evidence so far concerns yet another disease—cancer.

Adding Spice to Your Life

Like other spices, turmeric contains a bouquet of cancer-fighting compounds. The main one in turmeric is the yellow pigment *curcumin,* which makes turmeric—and hence curry—yellow. The compound is not well absorbed from the intestines into the rest of the body. But that's OK. The upside is that a lot of curcumin stays in the gastrointestinal tract, where it appears to fight colon polyps and possibly colon cancer, one of the most common cancers in the United States.

Curcumin's anti-cancer action derives in part from its antioxidant strength. But its anti-inflammatory potential is equally important. That's because inflammation leads to the release of damaging substances that can turn on cell proliferation. But Drs. Andrew Dannenberg and Kotha Subbaramaiah of New York Presbyterian Hospital-Cornell Medical Center have shown that curcumin can block the release of these substances by turning off a gene called cyclooxygenase-2, or COX-2, which makes the inflammatory COX-2 enzymes. "COX-2 inhibitors are one of the hottest areas of research in cancer prevention today, especially colon cancer," says Dannenberg. Other COX-2 inhibitors, such as the arthritis drugs Celebrex and Vioxx, also fight damaging inflammation. "But unlike Celebrex and Vioxx, which inhibit the activity of COX-2 enzymes, curcumin prevents their production in the first place," says Dannenberg.

That can only be good news—and for many conditions other than colon polyps and cancer. Christian Jobin, a research professor of medicine at the University of North Carolina, Chapel Hill, is examining whether curcumin can also be used to fight other intestinal ailments, such as colitis and inflammatory bowel syndrome. The early results look promising.

What's in a Name?

Despite the name, there is no curcumin in the spice cumin. (You can tell at a glance that it doesn't have that bright golden hue.) But cumin contains plenty of other intriguing phytochemicals. It derives its flavor from a complex brew of compounds, including pinene, cineole, terpineol, limonene, and cuminaldehyde. All have beneficial properties. But perhaps the most interesting compound of all is *farnesol,* which is found in high concentrations in cumin. It's a terpenoid that contributes flavor—and possibly much more.

Pamela Crowell, associate professor of biology at Indiana University-Purdue University Indianapolis, has found that farnesol is very effective in suppressing pancreatic cancer in hamsters. That's probably because it encourages apoptosis, or programmed cell death, among abnormal cells. "It can inhibit the growth of tumors, and even cause them to regress or disappear," says Crowell. "It's probably the most potent of the fifty terpenoids we've tested so far for pancreatic cancer, including perillyl alcohol and *d*-limonene." A synthetic derivative of farnesol appears even more effective in animal tests. If a farnesol-related drug could one day treat pancreatic tumors in people, that would be an incredible advance. "There is virtually no hope for patients diagnosed with pancreatic cancer," says Crowell. "The best chemotherapy prolongs life by only months."

Of course, one cannot achieve chemotherapeutic effects by adding a dash of cumin to dinner every now and then. But Charles Elson, professor of nutritional sciences at the University of Wisconsin College of Agriculture and Life Sciences, believes that small amounts of phytochemicals also have a protective effect when they're combined. "Our interest is in showing you don't need lots of any single terpene," says Elson. "If you eat a huge variety, the effects are additive or synergistic." Variety, it seems, really is the spice of life.

GREEN

4

"[Avocado growers] denied publicly and indignantly the insidious, slanderous rumors that avocados were aphrodisiac. Sales immediately mounted."
                        —Waverly Root (on an avocado publicity campaign),
                                                    Food (1980)

MORE THAN ANY OTHER HUE, green is the color of life. Who can imagine a living planet without green? Its return in the springtime heralds the promise of forsythia, lavender, and sweet-scented flowers. The yellow-green of spring yields to the rich, ripe fullness of the summer, with the fruits and crops we need to nourish and sustain us. A green planet is a healthy planet. And all of this is made possible by the green pigment chlorophyll.

Life as we know it would not exist without chlorophyll. Thanks to chlorophyll, green grasses, trees, and plants can use the sun's energy to generate food. Through photosynthesis, they convert carbon dioxide and water into carbohydrates, and in the process they release oxygen into the atmosphere. Without carbohydrates and oxygen, where would we be today? The preferred fuel of the brain and the body is carbohydrates, and oxygen keeps us breathing. In a very real sense, chlorophyll sustains life on this earth.

The main reason to eat greens isn't to consume chlorophyll, however, but to tap into the extraordinary bounty of life-giving phytochemicals that are packed into these foods. Any way you look at it, green means life.

SPINACH

Spinach at a Glance

- Pigments: chlorophyll, beta-carotene, lutein
- Other phytochemicals: glutathione, alpha-lipoic acid, D-glucaric acid, saponins, patuletin, spinacetin, spinatoside
- Serving size: one cup, chopped, raw
- Vitamins and minerals per serving: A (75% of the Daily Value), C (27% DV), K (400% DV), folate (27% DV), potassium (9% DV), riboflavin (6% DV), B_6 (5% DV), thiamin (3% DV), iron (4% DV), calcium (6% DV), zinc (2% DV)
- Fiber per serving: 6% DV
- ORAC score: 1,260

When was the last time your eye doctor gave you nutritional advice? Probably never, if he's the average doctor. But then, Steven Pratt is not the ordinary ophthalmologist. Pratt tells his patients at the Scripps Clinic in La Jolla, California, just what they need to be doing if they want to avoid eye troubles in old age. At the top of the list? "Eat spinach," he says. "Eat it raw. Eat it cooked. Eat it any way you can find to eat it. I call it the king of vegetables." That's because spinach is one of the richest (and most palatable) sources of the yellow-orange carotenoid lutein. Lutein is one of the main antioxidants in the eye. And since the body uses lutein to manufacture yet another antioxidant, the carotenoid zeaxanthin, you get two for the price of one. "I tell all my patients that spinach is one of the best things you can eat for your eyes," says Pratt. "I'm sure I've increased per capita consumption of spinach in San Diego County."

The Eyes Have It

As Pratt is quick to inform his patients, the lutein in spinach plays a crucial role in preventing age-related macular degeneration, the leading cause of blindness in the elderly. This disease results from the deterioration of the macula, the super-sensitive central region of the retina. When the macula goes, it takes the center of a person's field of vision along with it. In the less serious "dry" form,

THE BEST SOURCE OF YELLOW AND ORANGE IS GREEN!

Strange as it may seem, the best sources of yellow-orange lutein are not yellow vegetables, but green ones. But this shouldn't be a surprise if you recall why plants make carotenoids in the first place. These antioxidant pigments protect against free radicals that are generated when sunlight strikes chlorophyll. The darker the green vegetable, the more chlorophyll it contains—and the greater its need for antioxidant protection. Bottom line: Eat that sprig of parsley on your plate! It's good for more than decoration. Here are the top sources of lutein.

Food	Lutein
Kale	21.9*
Collard greens	16.3
Spinach	12.6
Watercress	12.5
Parsley	10.2
Mustard greens	9.9
Okra	6.8
Red peppers	6.8
Romaine lettuce	5.7
Broccoli	1.9
Brussels sprouts	1.3
Yellow corn	0.9

*measured in milligrams per 100 grams (about 3.5 ounces) of food
Source: USDA-NCI Carotenoid Database

macular degeneration may affect only the ability to perceive sharp, detailed images. But once the disease progresses to the devastating "wet" form, people can no longer see what is directly in front of them. Imagine turning your eyes toward a loved one or a loud noise and seeing nothing there but a blank spot, with only a bit of fuzzy peripheral vision around the outside. That is macular degeneration. Pratt watched his mother struggle with the disease.

She passed away at 91, but was declared legally blind at 75. "She was healthy as a horse, but she couldn't see, couldn't go places," he says.

To understand why lutein and zeaxanthin are so important to the eye, start with their color. These pigments appear yellow because they absorb blue light—and it's blue light that is most damaging to the macula. (Ultraviolet light would be equally harmful, but it is generally filtered out by the lens and cornea before it can reach the back of the eye.) The problem with blue light, says Pratt, is that it generates oxygen radicals. With time, these free radicals degrade the light-sensitive rods and cones that enable you to see. Free-radical damage also leads to the buildup of cellular debris that impedes vision. If you wear sunglasses with amber lenses, you will filter out some of this damaging blue light. But to absorb the remaining blue rays that sneak through, your eye needs lutein and zeaxanthin, too. They are the *only* carotenoids in the macula. "Think of them as internal sunglasses," says Pratt.

The first scientist to demonstrate the effectiveness of lutein and zeaxanthin in fighting macular degeneration was Dr. Johanna Seddon of Harvard. In 1994, she published a landmark study in the prestigious *Journal of the American Medical Association* showing that participants who ate the most carotenoid-rich foods decreased their risks of macular degeneration by a stunning 43 percent. Seddon noticed the greatest reduction in those who ate a lot of spinach and collard greens—both of them loaded with lutein and zeaxanthin.

Note: High spinach consumption is important for everyone, but it is especially critical for three high-risk groups—women, because their eyes do not absorb lutein as efficiently as men's; people with blue eyes, because a light-colored iris seems to allow more damaging light to penetrate to the back of the eye; and those with a family history of macular degeneration. All three are more likely to develop the disease.

Seeing the Light
Even if you're not at special risk for macular degeneration, that's no reason to slack off on your lutein. It could make all the difference to

more subtle measures of vision, too. As we age, the rods and cones in our eyes become less sensitive to green and blue light and more sensitive to glare. "You have a hard time seeing in dim lighting," says Billy Hammond, professor of vision science at the University of Georgia. "Things like glare kill you when you drive at night." But dense quantities of lutein and zeaxanthin in the macula can help ward off both problems. Hammond compared normal, healthy men and women in their 60s and 70s to a younger group in their 20s and 30s. Despite advanced age, the older folks with the most lutein and zeaxanthin in their maculas had "very youthful vision," Hammond reports. They didn't necessarily have 20/20 eyesight—but their eyes maintained all the responsivity of young eyes. Just one cup of spinach three or four times a week can make a dramatic difference. "But that's four times more than most people eat," he says.

Stopping Tunnel Vision

Lutein could also help fight an inherited disease called retinitis pigmentosa, in which the rods and cones near the outer portion of the retina deteriorate. The result is the loss of peripheral vision. As the disease progresses, the deterioration gradually spreads throughout the retina—both toward the center and out to the periphery. "As the visual field shrinks, you get tunnel vision and eventually blindness," says Gislin Dagnelie, assistant professor of ophthalmology at the Wilmer Eye Institute of Johns Hopkins University.

Dagnelie coordinated a six-month pilot study, in which 16 members of an online support group took lutein supplements and closely monitored their vision, using self-administered tests that Dagnelie devised. Twelve of the participants showed significant improvements in visual acuity and peripheral vision in as little as three to six weeks; those with blue eyes appeared to show stronger improvements than those with dark eyes. "What we don't know yet is whether lutein supplements will slow the progression of the disease over the long term," says Dagnelie. He's now starting a year-long trial that, unlike the original study, is placebo controlled.

Stop Cataracts, Too

Lutein and zeaxanthin are found in other parts of the eye, too, including the crystalline lens. All light entering the eye is filtered through this lens. Over a lifetime, however, sun exposure and free-radical damage from UV light degrade its proteins. A cloudy film, or cataract, develops over this crucial part of the eye, making it difficult to see clearly. Because the lens does not replace old cells with new ones, the damaged cells are there for life. "That makes it all the more important to give them as much antioxidant protection as possible," says Hammond. "Lutein and zeaxanthin are the only carotenoids in the lens, just as they are the only carotenoids in the macula."

Apparently as a result of diet, people differ dramatically in how much of these pigments they have in their eyes. These differences can translate into different rates of cataracts. In one recent Harvard study, 77,466 nurses over age 45 were followed for 12 years. Overall, those nurses who ate the most lutein and zeaxanthin had 22 percent fewer cataract surgeries. But those who dined on two especially lutein-rich foods—spinach and kale—were able to reduce their risks still more. Women who ate spinach two or more times a week (especially cooked spinach) lowered their risks by 30 to 38 percent. Those nurses who served up kale once or more a week slashed their risks by 40 percent.

Similarly, a companion study of 36,000 male physicians found that doctors who consumed the most lutein-rich foods had 19 percent fewer cataract surgeries. Among the men, broccoli and spinach were most consistently associated with a lower risk.

The Complete Eye-Saver Program

Spinach is not the only food that ophthalmologist Steven Pratt tells people to eat in order to ward off cataracts and macular degeneration. He also recommends a big bowl of blueberries every day, because of their potent antioxidants. And he urges patients to consume cold-water fish, such as salmon and tuna, a few times a week to benefit from their vital omega-3 oils.

But eye health, like health in general, depends on more than diet alone. That's why Pratt also makes the following recommendations:

- Avoid tobacco. "Smoking is the most preventable cause of cataracts and macular degeneration," he says. "There is a lot

of research showing that it reduces macular pigment density."
- If you drink alcohol, consume no more than six drinks a week if you're a man or three if you're a woman. "Alcohol is an oxidative stressor," he says. "It forms free radicals and lowers the blood's levels of lutein and zeaxanthin."
- Exercise regularly. "Exercise stimulates blood flow," says Pratt. "To nourish an organ, you need blood flow to bring in nutrients and carry out the bad guys."
- Wear sunglasses and hats on sunny days to reduce the amount of light entering the eye. If possible, buy sunglasses with amber lenses to filter out blue light. That will help protect against macular degeneration. For cataract protection, make sure the lenses also filter out ultraviolet light.

All of these elements together are necessary. That's why lutein supplements alone won't protect your vision as you age. "It's the sum total," says Pratt. "Lutein's fabulous. You can't do without it, but it's not the whole story. The *whole story* is the whole story."

What About Chlorophyll?
In a book about colorful foods, it's hard to ignore the quintessential green pigment, chlorophyll. In conventional and alternative medicine, it's used mainly as a breath freshener and skin deodorizer. It also slows the growth of bacteria and may have a mild antiseptic effect. Those are modest but useful properties.

New research, however, indicates, that chlorophyll may do far more. In a number of studies, it has been shown to be a reasonably good inhibitor of cancer—at least in mice and rainbow trout. It appears to work by latching onto potent carcinogens in the digestive tract and preventing their absorption into the body. These carcinogens include the heterocyclic amines (which cause colorectal cancer) and aflatoxin (which has been implicated in liver cancer). George Bailey of Oregon State University and Thomas Kensler of Johns Hopkins are currently conducting a study on a small peninsula near the mouth of the Yangtze River in China, where aflatoxin probably accounts for the exceptionally high incidence of liver cancer. For four months, the scientists gave 180 participants either placebo tablets or 100 milligrams of chlorophyllin—a water-soluble derivative of chlorophyll—three times a day to see if the chlorophyllin could help prevent cancer. The results aren't in yet. But even if we don't have the final word on chlorophyll, we still have every reason to fill our diets with greens, given their wealth of other life-sustaining phytonutrients.

Beyond the Eyes

Popeye used to gulp down spinach by the can. The theory was that its iron would build his muscles. That only goes to show why we shouldn't learn our nutrition lessons from cartoons. In fact, half the iron in spinach is bound to oxalic acid, making it unavailable for our bodies' general use. Most of spinach's calcium, too, is bound by oxalic acid. But no matter. Popeye was benefiting in many other ways from his heaping helpings of spinach. Those green leaves contain a gold mine of nutrients, including beta-carotene, potassium, and vitamin C. Recent research has also identified a number of novel cancer-fighting flavonoids that appear to be unique to spinach, including patuletin, spinacetin, and spinatoside.

Spinach is also an excellent source of folate. That's hardly surprising when you consider that this B vitamin derives its name from the Latin word *folium*, meaning "leaf." Folate (or "folic acid," as the man-made version is called) has received a lot of press in recent years for helping pregnant women prevent neural-tube defects such as spina bifida in their babies. But it's not just women of childbearing age who need it. Folate also appears to play a major role in preventing heart disease. That's because it helps your body dispose of a troublesome amino acid called homocysteine, which seems to make blood vessels susceptible to damage. Many scientists now rank homocysteine alongside cholesterol and smoking as a risk factor for heart disease. As if this isn't bad enough, high homocysteine is now being implicated in everything from cerebrovascular disease to osteoporosis. A recent study even found that cells in a test tube aged faster in the presence of homocysteine. Because homocysteine levels increase as we age, it's doubly important to eat your spinach as you get older.

Spinach is also one of the leading sources of vitamin K. Although scientists do not know as much about vitamin K as the other vitamins, they know that it helps at least 12 proteins in the body to carry out their functions. These specific proteins are found in blood, bones, arterial walls, and even the brain. Scientists have shown that without it, blood doesn't clot properly when we cut ourselves. Now they are finding that it is important for healthy bones, too. "A number of studies show that older women who eat lots of vitamin K have denser bones—and fewer hip fractures," says nutritionist Sarah Booth of the Human Nutrition Research Center on Aging at Tufts. "Spinach is one of the primary sources of vitamin K in this country." The simple rule of thumb, according to Booth, is this: "The greener the plant, the more vitamin K it contains, because vitamin K is part of the photosynthetic system." (One caveat: If you are taking the blood-thinning drug Coumadin, do not increase your intake of vitamin K. The vitamin interferes with Coumadin, making it less effective.)

Antioxidant Muscle

Spinach also contains two important antioxidants—*glutathione* and *alpha-lipoic acid*. These are the two most important antioxidants in the body, according to Lester Packer, professor emeritus of molecular cell biology at the University of California at Berkeley and author of *The Antioxidant Miracle*. We do not often hear about these antioxidants, because the body can manufacture them itself. But the body does not always make enough to meet its needs, especially as we age.

Glutathione is the main antioxidant in cells. It's found in the watery interior of cells, where it protects DNA from oxidation. "Maintaining a high level of glutathione is critical for life," says Packer. "In fact, low glutathione levels are a marker for death at any age." Packer calls glutathione "nature's master antioxidant." But it plays many other crucial roles in the body, too—detoxifying pollutants and carcinogens, maintaining a healthy liver, boosting the immune system, aiding healthy cell replication, repairing damaged DNA, and reducing chronic inflammation. If Packer's suspicions prove correct, it may even help prolong life.

Our bodies make most of their glutathione from three amino acids that are abundant in foods. But glutathione also comes ready-made in vegetables and fruits like spinach, asparagus, avocados, and strawberries. Only a small portion of our total glutathione comes directly from these foods, but that doesn't mean that it's unimportant. "It gets absorbed by the cells in the mouth and pharynx, which use it to support detoxification reactions," says biochemist Dean Jones of the Emory University School of Medicine. "In fact, these cells don't synthesize as much glutathione as other cells in the body, so they need the glutathione in fruits and vegetables." In one of his many trials on the antioxidant, Jones studied 1,830 people and found that those who ate the most glutathione-rich foods had just half the cancers of the mouth and pharynx as those who ate the least—but only if the foods were eaten raw. "Stir-fried vegetables won't lose much, but if you boil vegetables the way your grandmother did, there will be no glutathione left at all," he says.

Nature's Superantioxidant

The other way to boost your glutathione levels is to consume alpha-lipoic acid—and there happens to be a small amount of that in spinach, too. Alpha-lipoic acid increases glutathione by helping cells absorb a critical amino acid that is needed to make it.

But that's not the only reason you need alpha-lipoic acid. Packer calls it a "superantioxidant." Most other antioxidants are soluble in either watery portions of the body (such as the blood) or fatty tissues (such as cell membranes). Alpha-lipoic acid is soluble in both, meaning that it can help defend every type of substance in the body against oxidative assaults. It guards against stroke, heart attacks, and cataracts. It strengthens memory. It turns off genes that can accelerate aging and cause cancer. And it helps the body break down sugar for energy production.

As with glutathione, the body makes the bulk of its alpha-lipoic acid from common constituents of the diet. But foods like spinach, broccoli, tomatoes, potatoes, peas, and Brussels sprouts also deliver small amounts. Of these, spinach is the best.

WHERE TO FIND "NATURE'S MASTER ANTIOXIDANT"
Our bodies make most of their glutathione from common amino acids in the diet. But about 5 percent of glutathione comes directly from food. Here are the best sources:

Food	Glutathione
Asparagus	28.3*
Avocados	27.7
Potatoes, boiled w/ skin	13.6
Spinach, raw	12.2
Okra	12.0
Strawberries	9.9
Grapefruit, white	7.9
Peaches	7.4
Oranges	7.3
Cantaloupe	6.9
Watermelon	6.6

*measured in milligrams per 100 grams (about 3.5 ounces) of food
Source: Dean Jones, Emory University School of Medicine

How to Clean Your Spinach and Eat It, Too

Washing spinach can be tedious. But if that's all that's standing between you and a large spinach salad, here's a simple tip: Buy a nice, fresh bunch of spinach with the stems on. When you get home, fill a large bowl with cold water and add a couple table-spoons of vinegar. Holding the spinach by the stems, immerse the leaves in the water, and swirl them around the bowl several times vigorously. The sand and grit will come right off and sink to the bottom.

Another simple solution is to buy packages of prewashed baby spinach.

When it comes to preparing spinach, there is much debate over whether one should cook the greens or not. There is no sim-ple answer. Cooking degrades folate and vitamin C. On the other hand, it frees up the carotenoids, particularly beta-carotene.

Lutein becomes more available, too, although it is more bioavailable than beta-carotene in the first place. Bottom line: Eat your spinach raw sometimes; eat it cooked on other occasions. When you do cook it, try to steam it lightly or cook it for as short a time as possible. Chopping and puréeing are other good ways to prepare spinach and free up the carotenoids at the same time.

> QUICK 'N' EASY
>
> Are you still trying to figure out how to work spinach into your diet? It's wonderful in salads. For a particularly delicious variation on the standard spinach salad, use tarragon vinegar in the dressing. Top the salad with toasted almonds, mandarin oranges, sliced mushrooms, and fresh tarragon.

AVOCADOS

Avocados at a Glance

- Pigments: chlorophyll, beta-carotene, lutein
- Other phytochemicals: glutathione, beta-sitosterol, p-coumaric acid, chlorogenic acid, ferulic acid, caffeic acid, syringic acid, vanillic acid, gallic acid
- Serving size: one-half medium avocado
- Vitamins and minerals per serving: A (18% of the Daily Value), C (20% DV), folate (20% DV), B_6 (20% DV), niacin (15% DV), thiamin (10% DV), riboflavin (10% DV), E (13% DV), potassium (20% DV), magnesium (13% DV), zinc (5% DV)
- Fiber per serving: 33% DV
- ORAC score: 782

In 1519, when Hernán Cortés landed in Mexico, he found a fruit that he had never seen before. The Aztecs called it the *ahuacatl*. Dark green and rough on the outside, it was rich and velvety smooth on the inside. The people of the New World had numerous uses for this fruit. They made a paste out of it that was the

Rogaine of its day. They created ointments that were supposed to delay old age. They even used it as an aphrodisiac, no doubt because of its suggestive shape. (*Ahuacatl* also means "testicle." Just think of the image in people's minds when they named the avocado tree the "testicle tree"!)

To the Europeans, the more defining characteristic of the avocado was its creamy texture. As the conquistadors' chronicler wrote, the avocado is "similar to butter and of very good taste." To this day, that smooth, fat-laden richness is both the attraction of this fruit and the reason why dieters avoid it like a triple fudge sundae. Admittedly, avocados do have an exceptionally high fat content for a fruit—accounting for more than 80 percent of its calories. That's why you shouldn't devour a whole bowl of guacamole by yourself. On the other hand, two-thirds of the fat in avocados is the "good," monounsaturated variety that does not raise blood cholesterol. In fact, avocados can even help lower cholesterol and triglycerides, a type of blood fat that may contribute to heart disease.

The "Green" Way to Help Lower Cholesterol

Avocados contain another substance that helps lower cholesterol, too. It's called *beta-sitosterol,* and it's one of the phytosterols—the equivalent in plants of cholesterol in animals. Because it is so similar in structure to cholesterol, beta-sitosterol competes with cholesterol for absorption into the body—and wins. The result is lower cholesterol in the bloodstream. The margarine replacements Take Control and Benecol incorporate phytosterols or related stanols—and both can help reduce cholesterol.

Beta-sitosterol does something else interesting. It appears to inhibit excessive cell division, which may help prevent cancer cell growth. That's not surprising, really. Cholesterol is essential for forming cell membranes. If phytosterols are blocking cholesterol absorption, there is less cholesterol available—and cancer cells cannot proliferate without the materials to form new membranes. Phytosterols not only reduce the supply of cellular building materials but also seem to affect the signaling process that lets cells know when to replicate and when to die. In both animal studies and lab tests, Atif Awad, director of the nutrition program at the

State University of New York at Buffalo, has found that beta-sitosterol helps reduce cancer.

And that's not all. Because phytosterols also inhibit the division of smooth muscle cells in arteries and veins, they may fight atherosclerosis, says Awad. "If you prevent cell proliferation there, you control the development of plaques."

Avocados are one of the best sources of beta-sitosterol, along with oils, nuts, and seeds.

NIX CHOLESTEROL—BOOST PHYTOSTEROLS INSTEAD
The leading sources of beta-sitosterol are nuts, oils, and legumes. But among fruits and vegetables, avocados are tops, by far.

Food	Beta-sitosterol
Peanut butter	135*
Cashews	130
Almonds	122
Peas	106
Kidney beans	91
Avocados	76
Oranges	17
Brussels sprouts	17
Sweet cherries	12
Cauliflower	12
Onions	12
Bananas	11
Apples	11

*measured in milligrams per 100 grams (about 3.5 ounces) of food
Sources: Atif Awad, SUNY Buffalo (peanut butter); David Kritchevsky, Wistar Institute (all other foods)

Topping the Charts

Avocados contain plenty of other good stuff, too. A study by Paul Lachance at Rutgers University found that avocados were one of the top ten nutrient-dense foods. Ounce for ounce, he discovered, avocados topped the charts for folate, potassium, magnesium, and vitamin E among fruits. They are also an excellent source of B vitamins and fiber. And as if that isn't bounty enough, they include a long list of cancer-fighting phytochemicals, including *p*-coumaric acid, chlorogenic acid, ferulic acid, and gallic acid, along with more ready-made glutathione than any other fruit or vegetable except asparagus. Glutathione, as we've already noted, is one of the body's most essential antioxidants.

All this goodness doesn't come free, though. Ounce for ounce, the avocado has more calories than any other fruit. A whole avocado racks up 300 calories—and you know how easy it is to eat a whole avocado. That means that if you start adding avocados to your diet, you need to subtract calories elsewhere.

QUICK 'N' EASY

Because of their nutty, creamy texture, avocados used to be known as "poor man's butter." You didn't have to be wealthy enough to own cows, just a few trees in the backyard. Even today some people use these so-called butter pears in lieu of actual butter—although the goal these days is better nutrition rather than cost savings. Elizabeth Pivonka, president of the Produce for Better Health Foundation, says that avocado on sandwiches gives the "mouth feel" of mayonnaise, but with a bounty of vitamins, minerals, and phytonutrients. Pivonka also advocates using guacamole instead of salad dressing. "My family's motto is, once you've tried it, you're hooked," she says.

Care and Handling of Avocados

To ripen avocados, place them in a paper bag with a banana or tomato. (In a plastic bag, they will not ripen at all.) Avocados are ready to eat when they feel slightly soft to the touch. At that point, if you don't plan to use them right away, move them to the refrigerator. They will keep there for a few days.

Once avocados have been cut open, they brown like apples.

There is a myth that putting the avocado pit in the guacamole will keep it fresh. Not so. The best way to prevent it from oxidizing is to squeeze lemon or lime juice over it. Alternatively, you can cover the bowl with plastic wrap that is pressed down against the guacamole to keep the oxygen out.

ASPARAGUS

Asparagus is a no-nonsense plant. Other vegetables may expend energy growing splendid stalks or showy vines. But asparagus just sends its efficient little spears straight up out of the ground. No muss, no fuss. It takes a couple of years for an asparagus root to develop fully, but once it does, it produces a new spear every few days. Within just three to five days, a new one is 10 inches high and ready for handpicking. "On a warm day, you can almost watch the asparagus grow," says asparagus breeder Brian Benson. "The fastest I've seen them grow is eight inches in a day—a third of an inch an hour."

Asparagus doesn't mess around when it comes to nutrition, either. It zooms to the top of the charts, with a mighty 33 percent of the daily value of folate. It also has a good supply of other vitamins and minerals. And as for phytochemicals, asparagus is the number-one source of ready-made glutathione in our diets. It also contains a flavonoid called *rutin*, which works with vitamin C to strengthen capillary walls. At just four calories a spear, how can you go wrong?

Here's a quick summary of the good stuff in asparagus:

- Pigments: chlorophyll, beta-carotene, lutein, anthocyanins (various forms of cyanidin)
- Other phytochemicals: glutathione, rutin, saponins, lignans
- Serving size: one-half cup, or six spears
- Vitamins and minerals per serving: A (10% of the Daily Value), C (17% DV), folate (33% DV), thiamin (7% DV), B$_6$ (6% DV), riboflavin (6% DV), niacin (5% DV), E (4% DV), potassium (4% DV), iron (4% DV)
- Fiber per serving: 6% DV
- ORAC score: 1,200 (measured by Brunswick Labs)

ARTICHOKES

Artichokes at a Glance
- Pigments: chlorophyll, beta-carotene
- Other phytochemicals: silymarin, cynarin, chlorogenic acid, caffeic acid, inulin
- Serving size: one 12-ounce artichoke
- Vitamins and minerals per serving: C (10% of the Daily Value), folate (10% DV), magnesium (10% DV), potassium (5% DV), niacin (4% DV), B_6 (4% DV), iron (4% DV), thiamin (2% DV), riboflavin (2% DV), zinc (2% DV), copper (2% DV), pantothenic acid (2% DV)
- Fiber per serving: 16% DV
- ORAC score: not available

The late sportswriter Pete Axthelm once wrote a piece in *Newsweek* about the difficulties of getting dates when you are, as he put it, a "balding, cigar-smoking sportswriter who enjoys hanging out until closing time in smoky saloons." It was a curiously charming article. But perhaps the most memorable line in it was a quote from one of his lady friends, a self-proclaimed expert on bad boyfriends. "Love," this woman declared, "can be like eating an artichoke. All that work to go through all those layers, and then there's so little there."

Well, that may be true of love in some cases. But it's worth taking the trouble to get to an artichoke heart. As you work your way through all those layers, you'll get a hefty serving of vitamin C, magnesium, folate, and fiber. You'll also get a variety of heart-healthy phytochemicals. In a recent German study, 143 patients with high cholesterol were given either 1,800 milligrams of dry artichoke extract or a placebo every day for six weeks. At the end, those taking the extract had reduced their total cholesterol by 18 percent on average and had reduced their "bad" LDL cholesterol by 23 percent, resulting in a better overall ratio of HDL to LDL—nearly as great an improvement as with medication. At least part of the effect was probably due to a compound called *cynarin,* which increases the liver's production of bile. Bile in turn helps the body remove cholesterol.

"As Good As It Gets"

As a bonus, the artichoke heart will give you small amounts of a group of flavonoids that are collectively known as *silymarin*. Unless you dine on milk thistle, which few people do, artichokes are likely to be the only place that you'll find silymarin in your diet. It's worth eating some every now and then. "This is a miracle agent," says cancer biologist Rajesh Agarwal of the AMC Cancer

QUICK 'N' EASY

The quickest way to fix artichokes is to savor marinated artichoke hearts straight out of the jar. They also make a great antipasto dish, with roasted red peppers, prosciutto, and fresh mozarella.

We'd be lying, though, if we told you that there was a quick 'n' easy way to prepare these vegetables fresh. They take so much time to cook that, in some parts of the world, they are favorites of the International Slow Food Movement—a grass-roots movement dedicated to the leisurely pleasures of good eating, with special emphasis on regional specialties and organic produce.

The best way to cook fresh artichokes is to cut off the stem at the bottom. Remove the tough outer leaves. Then slice an inch from the top of the remaining leaves. Stand the artichokes upright in the bottom of a pot and fill it with one to two inches of water. Bring the water to a boil; then turn down the heat and simmer, covered, for 45 minutes. Add more water, if necessary. When you can pull out a leaf easily, the artichokes are done.

To eat the cooked artichokes, pull off the leaves one at a time and dip them in a low-fat sauce (such as the Roasted Red Pepper Dressing on page 238). Scrape off the soft pulp at the bottom of each leaf with your teeth. There will be more pulp on leaves closer to the center. When you approach the end, you will find a fuzzy part called the choke. This is not edible. Beneath the choke, however, is the prize—the heart, which is delicious. Enjoy!

Research Center in Denver. "In Europe and Asia, it's been used for centuries in the form of milk thistle seeds to treat liver toxicity—hepatitis, cirrhosis, and alcohol-related problems."

As Agarwal's research shows, silymarin is also a major cancer-fighting compound that functions in many ways at once. It's a strong antioxidant and a potent anti-inflammatory. It ratchets up detoxification enzymes. It stifles uncontrolled replication by encouraging a process called cell differentiation. It even inhibits the internal cell signaling that tells a cell to keep growing. With all these functions to its credit, it certainly ought to fight cancer, and that is precisely what Agarwal is finding in animal experiments.

He started by using silymarin topically on skin cancers in mice. The results were startling. "It reduced the number of mice who developed cancers by seventy-five percent," says Agarwal. Those that did develop tumors had 92 percent fewer cancers, and the tumor size in them was 97 percent smaller. "In cancer research, that's as good as it gets," he says. He has since begun giving the animals silymarin orally to see if it can prevent prostate tumors, too. So far, it seems to be working. Mice given silymarin remain cancer-free far longer than untreated mice, and when cancers do form, they are just one-fifth the size of cancers in untreated mice.

Unfortunately, you won't get enough silymarin from artichokes to guarantee a cancer-free existence. But an artichoke every now and then clearly can't hurt. It's just one more weapon in your disease-fighting arsenal.

BROCCOLI

Broccoli at a Glance
- Pigments: chlorophyll, lutein, beta-carotene
- Other phytochemicals: glucoraphanin (sulforaphane), glucobrassicin (indole-3-carbinol), glucoerucin, glucoiberin, D-glucaric acid, caffeic acid, quercetin, alpha-lipoic acid, lignans
- Serving size: one-half cup, chopped, raw
- Vitamins and minerals per serving: A (14% of the Daily Value), C (68% DV), K (81% DV), E (7% DV), folate (8%

DV), potassium (4% DV), phosphorus (3% DV), calcium
(2% DV), iron (2% DV)
- Fiber per serving: 5% DV
- ORAC score: 890

Broccoli traces its roots (literally) to the shores of the sunny
Mediterranean Sea, where it used to grow wild along the coast. It
was the Italians who first plucked and tamed the vegetable, which
they enthusiastically embraced as part of their cooking. Other cultures eventually adopted broccoli and even transplanted it to
America. George Washington and Thomas Jefferson both grew it
in their kitchen gardens—a welcome contrast to a more recent
president, also named George, who famously declared in 1992,
"I'm president of the United States, and I'm not going to eat any
more broccoli."

Despite the horticultural experiments of Washington and Jefferson, it was not until the 1920s that Italian immigrants really
began popularizing the vegetable in America. Consumption
increased eightfold between then and 1990. In the last decade, it's
jumped another 80 percent, thanks largely to news about broccoli's extraordinary health benefits.

Broccoli is truly a wonder, with its rich store of protective
flavonoids, terpenes, and phenolics. As if this weren't bounty
enough, it also delivers an amazing series of cancer-preventing
compounds called *isothiocyanates* and *indoles*. It's hard to beat
that combination for combating numerous diseases, especially
cancer. As food writers Jeannette Ferrary and Louise Fiszer have
said, "If people were attracted to what was good for them, movie
theaters would sell cartons of hot, buttered broccoli and ballfields
would specialize in broccoli on a bun with mustard and relish."

The Talalay Factor

If broccoli is enjoying a newfound popularity today, much of that
success is due to the work of one man, Dr. Paul Talalay of Johns
Hopkins University, who has unlocked some of the secrets of
broccoli's cancer-fighting powers. Talalay began his medical career
in the 1940s, when a diagnosis of cancer was almost always a
death sentence. In those days, doctors did not even tell their

patients they had the disease because the news would be too devastating. Then along came a scientist named Lee Wattenberg at the University of Minnesota. He demonstrated that two common antioxidants that were used to preserve food could help prevent cancer in animals. This was a huge breakthrough, says Talalay, and yet there was very little interest from the scientific community. "Wattenberg went from meeting to meeting talking about his results," says Talalay. "It was difficult to get a room small enough for those few who wanted to hear him." Such was the general disbelief in the possibilities of cancer prevention.

Talalay became a believer, though. He went on to show, through decades of research, that Wattenberg's antioxidants fought cancer not so much because of their antioxidant activity, but because they boosted levels of so-called phase 2 enzymes. These enzymes effectively rid the body of numerous carcinogens and pollutants. What's more, they protect against many types of cancer, not just one. The implications were huge. "If certain compounds in foods could boost our bodies' defenses against a variety of tumors, we wouldn't have to devise a specific strategy against each one," says Talalay. "A single strategy would protect against breast cancer and colon cancer, lung cancer, and stomach cancer." He set out to find the foods that contained the most "phase 2 enzyme inducers." Of course, you've guessed by now that the superstars turned out to be broccoli and its cruciferous cousins, including kale, cabbage, Brussels sprouts, cauliflower, turnips, and watercress.

At this point, though, Talalay still didn't know what compounds in the crucifers were boosting phase 2 enzymes. He singled out broccoli for intense scrutiny, largely because many people were already eating it. "We didn't want to get into a situation where we came up with a dietary recommendation for some exotic plant that nobody would eat anyway," he says.

In 1992, Talalay and his lab announced the discovery of a potent phase 2 inducer called *sulforaphane*. He quickly followed up that discovery with studies of sulforaphane in carcinogen-exposed rats. The results were stunning. Among those who received sulforaphane, the number of rats who developed mammary tumors was slashed by 60 percent. Moreover, in those animals who did develop cancers, the size of the tumors was cut by 75 percent.

Clamping Down on Cancer

The amazing thing about sulforaphane is how many different ways it helps battle cancer. As we've already noted, it increases the level of phase 2 enzymes. These enzymes are sort of like a local police force for the body. They grab trouble-causing carcinogens and handcuff them to something soluble like glutathione that can float away in the bloodstream. Then it's into the paddy wagon—or bloodstream, actually—which carries the troublemakers away to be flushed out of the body.

That alone is a powerful reason to seek out sulforaphane. But French scientists have recently discovered another. In lab tests with human colon-cancer cells, they've found that sulforaphane also causes cell cycle arrest and apoptosis (programmed cell death) in these abnormal cells. Both activities can help squelch the development of tumors.

And by boosting phase 2 enzymes, sulforaphane also helps the body fight oxidation. Talalay has recently discovered that these enzymes act as "indirect" antioxidants. They do not "quench" free radicals by giving up electrons, like vitamins E or C. But just as they directly link carcinogens to other molecules, they can inactivate oxygen radicals by hooking them to substances that the body then disposes of. They also boost production of glutathione, the master antioxidant, and increase levels of antioxidant-generating enzymes. "They may be the major antioxidant defenses of the cell," says Talalay. And because they are enzymes and don't get used up as they work, they remain in the body much longer than traditional antioxidants, which often last only hours. Together, these are some very powerful reasons to eat broccoli.

Have You Eaten Your BroccoSprouts Today?

The only problem with sulforaphane—as with most of the compounds in plants—is that it's impossible to predict how much is in any given specimen. The levels can vary wildly, depending on growing conditions. An average head of broccoli contains about 35,000 units of sulforaphane per gram. But the levels can range from 10,000 to 85,000. You, the customer, have no way of knowing just by looking.

But Paul Talalay made another interesting discovery. He found that three-day-old broccoli sprouts have at least 10 to 50 times more sulforaphane than mature broccoli. He also learned that he could consistently deliver the same amount by growing the sprouts under strict conditions. Together with Johns Hopkins University, he licensed the information to Brassica Protection Products LLC, which now supervises the production and marketing of trademarked BroccoSprouts. "We grow them like marijuana—indoors on tables under lights," Talalay jokes. The result is sprouts that deliver a whopping 200,000 units of sulforaphane per gram. They may be the only fresh food that guarantees a specified level of a phytochemical—and a potent cancer fighter, at that.

Indoles: Taming Estrogen

As impressive as sulforaphane is, it is only one of a family of similar compounds in cruciferous vegetables. Like the organosulfur compounds in onions and garlic, these substances are not actually formed until an insect—or a person, for that matter—bites or cuts into a crucifer. Then phytochemicals called *glucosinolates* are converted into a variety of sharp-tasting new compounds that keep insects at bay. If the new chemical contains sulfur, it's called an *isothiocyanate*. Sulforaphane is one of these. If the new chemical doesn't contain sulfur, it may be one of several compounds, including an *indole*. Broccoli has its share of these, too.

The most important indole in broccoli is *indole-3-carbinol*—or I3C, for short. Like sulforaphane, it appears to be a potent cancer fighter, but for different reasons. Sulforaphane stimulates detoxification enzymes. I3C can do this, too, to a lesser extent. But its main anti-cancer activity comes through its effects on estrogen. I3C works in two important ways.

First, it blocks estrogen receptors in breast cancer cells. Why does that matter? In order for any hormone such as estrogen to carry out its functions, it has to dock in a receptor on a cell's surface. The receptor is perfectly designed to accept that particular hormone, just like a lock and its key. But indole-3-carbinol can slip into estrogen receptors, too. By locking into these sites first, it can block estrogen. It's like a game of musical chairs where I3C sits down on the receptors before estrogen can reach them. Like the loser in musical chairs, estrogen is out of the game, at least for a while. That's important because many breast cancers are driven by estrogen. Only a fraction of the cells in a woman's breast have estrogen receptors, but the ones that do seem particularly vulnerable to cancer.

Second, indole-3-carbinol influences the balance of estrogens in our bodies. We're used to thinking of estrogen as just one substance, but actually there are numerous forms in our bodies at all times. (This goes for men, too, although their levels are much lower than women's.) Indole-3-carbinol drives production of a less potent estrogen that does not stimulate breast cancer and diminishes production of a more harmful form. According to a recent study by Jay Fowke at the University of South Carolina, just one serving of broccoli a day is enough to alter the balance favorably—although two or more servings are even better.

Indole-3-carbinol isn't only useful for preventing breast tumors. The more protective balance of estrogens also appears to fight human papilloma virus—a nasty bug that researchers believe increases the risks of cervical cancer, precancerous cervical lesions, and colon cancer. H. Leon Bradlow, professor of biochemistry at Weill Medical College of Cornell University in New York, has tested I3C on women with precancerous cervical lesions and has seen promising results. In a recent study, Bradlow and Dr. Maria Bell of the University of South Dakota Medical Center gave 30 women either a placebo or supplements of I3C for four months. In the test group, the lesions of half the women completely cleared up. In the placebo group, none did. If indole-3-carbinol in the end proves effective, it will be an important aid to treatment. "Surgery is only moderately helpful," says Bradlow. "You don't turn off the virus, so the condition comes back. With indole-3-carbinol, the virus stays dormant as long as you take the supplements."

Recently, supplement manufacturers have begun hawking I3C tablets. Once again, we would urge you to stay away from pills and eat broccoli instead. In certain lab conditions, large doses of purified I3C have actually increased cancer in animals. Bradlow has not observed this in human trials—and adds that a metabolite of I3C called diindolylmethane appears even safer. Still, he notes, "There is no such thing as a drug that is safe in unlimited quantities." Broccoli, by contrast, turns up over and over as a protective food—with the greatest benefits to those people who eat the most.

Still More Cancer Fighters

Broccoli has no lack of cancer-fighting chemicals. Yet another is D-glucaric acid. Glucaric acid helps detoxify a number of carcinogens, including polycyclic aromatic hydrocarbons, heterocyclic amines, and various nitrosamines. Studies in rats and mice have shown that glucaric acid inhibits tumors of the colon, mammary gland, liver, lung, skin, and bladder.

Broccoli also contains plenty of the yellow-orange pigment lutein. As you already know, lutein protects the eyes. Like the other major carotenoids, it may also inhibit cancer. Loïc Le Marchand of the University of Hawaii compared the diets of people in Fiji with those of three other South Pacific nations—Tahiti,

QUICK 'N' EASY

Broccoli consumption has nearly doubled in the last decade, thanks to revelations about its cancer-fighting prowess. And yet, there are still people who turn up their noses. For people who remain broccoli averse—not to mention folks who just want to boost their intake—here are some easy ways to sneak broccoli into the diet.

- Even finicky eaters love pizza—and broccoli happens to be a pizza-friendly topping. So are other veggies, like mushrooms, peppers, fresh garlic, and onions.
- Broccoli also goes well in pasta dishes, drenched in a tasty olive oil and garlic sauce, with zesty freshly grated Parmesan cheese on top. For the real broccoli haters, a marinara sauce does an even better job of disguising the flavor of broccoli, if not the texture.

You'll be glad to know that sulforaphane survives the cooking process. Try not to cook broccoli too long, though. And definitely don't boil it, or else nutrients will leach into the water. "Raw is best," says Jay Fowke of the University of South Carolina, "but many people find that steaming makes it more palatable."

New Caledonia, and the Cook Islands. He wanted to know why the Fijians have far less lung cancer than their fellow Pacific islanders, despite similar rates of smoking. Not surprisingly, he found that Fijians ate more vegetables in general—and more dark green vegetables in particular. They also had higher levels of lutein in their blood. According to Le Marchand, the data suggested an even greater role for lutein than for vitamin E, one of the top antioxidants.

Preventing Cancer Decades Ahead of Time

Put all this together, and you've got potent stuff. Paul Talalay remembers very clearly the day in 1971 when President Richard Nixon declared a national war on cancer. In the decades since then, scientists have made considerable progress. They've discovered oncogenes and tumor-suppressor genes. They've figured out the many steps in the lengthy and complex development of the disease. They've devised new treatments. But there's one thing they haven't done—reduce the incidence of cancer in any major way. And Talalay knows why. "Doctors focus on treating cancer in the short period when it is diagnosed," he says, "but they ignore the ten- to twenty-year period of cancer development." That's a decade or more in which the body's numerous repair mechanisms can step in and squelch a tumor for you—if you give your body the nutrients it needs to do the job. As Talalay says, it's much easier to prevent cancer in the first place than to treat the disease once it's taken hold.

Eat to Beat Heart Disease

OK, so cancer doesn't run in your family. Does that mean you can skip the broccoli? That depends. Are you concerned about heart disease? You should be. As Kirk Johnson wrote in the *New York Times,* "Most people do not sit down with statistical charts and decide on the basis of the evidence what specter of death or calamity should most fill them with dread. If they did, they would be pacing the floor at night over cardiovascular disease. Clogged arteries and bad hearts carry off nearly a million Americans a year, about as many as all other diseases and disasters combined."

Broccoli could turn out to be a very heart-friendly food, thanks in part to its lutein. You may recall a study in Chapter 3, comparing the heart-healthy residents of Toulouse with the not-so-healthy residents of Belfast. One of two major differences between the populations was that the robust citizens of Toulouse had far more lutein in their blood, thanks to their regular consumption of broccoli and Brussels sprouts.

Now James Dwyer, professor of preventive medicine at the Keck School of Medicine at the University of Southern California, has a new study suggesting that this was no coincidence. Dwyer followed 480 employees of a California utility company for 18 months and found that those with the highest levels of lutein in their blood showed the least amount of thickening in their carotid arteries over the study period. Carotid-artery thickness is a good indication of atherosclerosis, the underlying condition that leads to most heart attacks and strokes. The results? "Those in the top twenty percent of lutein levels showed almost no progression in atherosclerosis over the eighteen months," says Dwyer. "Those in the bottom twenty percent progressed five times faster."

The problem with observational studies like these is that they do not necessarily prove cause and effect. But Dwyer supported his findings with both animal and lab studies, which seem to confirm the human test results. In the animal trial, he took two types of mice that tend to develop high cholesterol levels and atherosclerosis. When their diets were supplemented with lutein, their blood vessels developed 40 to 50 percent fewer fatty deposits. Dwyer admits that he fed the animals "huge amounts" of lutein to achieve these effects. But he notes that since mice do not absorb lutein well, their blood levels were no higher than those of an average person.

Perhaps most intriguing of all, he obtained small segments from the aortas of heart-transplant patients and tested them in the lab. "If you put them in a petri dish and add LDL, you get an immune response," he says. In short, arterial walls that are filled with oxidized LDL attract white blood cells called monocytes, or macrophages. "When monocytes migrate into the artery wall, fill with oxidized LDL, and die in the artery wall, that is one of the first important steps in the development of atherosclerosis," says Dwyer. "The material inside them dumps out into the wall. Then the artery wall recruits more monocytes to clean that up. It's almost like an autoimmune response that just feeds on itself and builds into atherosclerosis." If one could block this immune response, one could vastly reduce the early development of atherosclerosis.

Dwyer's lab studies found that lutein helped do exactly that. "When we added lutein to these cells before adding the LDL, the cell wall didn't attract nearly as many monocytes," he says. That suggests that lutein is reducing heart disease not by quenching free radicals, but by altering the cell signaling that summons the white blood cells.

"A Very Potent Effect"

Broccoli's flavonoids may also benefit the cardiovascular system. A ten-year study of 34,492 postmenopausal women in Iowa found that deaths from heart disease were 38 percent lower among women in the top bracket of flavonoid intake. The only individual food that stood out as heart-protective in this trial was broccoli.

Another study that appeared recently in the *Journal of the American Medical Association* found that men and women who consumed five to six servings of fruits and vegetables a day lowered their risk of stroke by 31 percent. The strongest effect came from cruciferous vegetables—including broccoli, cauliflower, Brussels sprouts, and cabbage—followed by green leafy vegetables, citrus fruit, and citrus juice. "This is a very potent effect," says Dr. Ralph Sacco, associate chairman of neurology at Columbia University College of Physicians and Surgeons. "If it's validated by other studies, it may turn out that eating these foods can reduce stroke risk as much as the traditional methods of physical exercise and blood pressure control."

ALFALFA SPROUTS

BroccoSprouts are great, but that's no reason to ignore alfalfa sprouts. Alfalfa sprouts have one of the top ORAC scores—930. They're one of the leading sources of cancer-fighting D-glucaric acid. And along with such legumes as chickpeas and soybeans, they are among the best sources of *saponins*. These useful chemicals lower cholesterol by latching onto it in the digestive tract and carrying it right on through the system, without allowing it to be absorbed. "In simple terms, saponins are like natural detergents," explains Venket Rao, professor of nutrition at the University of Toronto. Think of your digestive tract as a greasy frying pan.

Rinsing that frying pan with water leaves an oily film behind, because no part of the water molecule is able to grab on to the oil molecule and carry it away. But once you add detergent, which can grab on to both oil and water, you begin to cut through the grease and move it on.

Believe it or not, this mechanism may have applications in the fight against cancer, too. Cell membranes contain many fatty components, including cholesterol. "The hypothesis is that saponins are able to attach to the cholesterol and break up membranes like detergents busting the greasy film in your frying pan," asserts Rao. Without their membranes intact, the cancer cells die. Fortunately, saponins do not have this effect on normal cells. "Since cancer cells have higher levels of cholesterol in the membrane, saponins have more binding sites and therefore a greater effect on cancer cells than normal cells," Rao explains. Saponins are not readily absorbed from the digestive tract into the bloodstream, so they appear to be useful mainly for combating colon cancer.

KALE, CABBAGE, WATERCRESS, AND BRUSSELS SPROUTS

As wonderful as broccoli is, it is just one of many cruciferous vegetables, including cabbage, kale, watercress, Brussels sprouts, cauliflower, and turnips. All of them appear to have cancer-fighting power. Which is the best? It's no more possible to answer this question than to say which of your children is the "best." Although they're related, they're all different—and all wonderful.

In the same way, the crucifers are clearly related, yet different and wonderful at the same time. Not all of them give you as much sulforaphane as broccoli does. But sulforaphane is just one of many isothiocyanates. There are also several cancer-fighting indoles in the crucifers, not to mention a number of carotenoids. The crucifers mix and match these beneficial compounds—one from column A, two from column B—as if they were items on the proverbial Chinese menu.

That is why you can't go wrong eating cruciferous vegetables—and also why it's good to eat a variety of them. "If you focus on one food, you can end up missing the benefits in others," says Dr. Henry Thompson, who heads up the Center for Nutrition in the Prevention of Disease at the AMC Cancer Research Center in Denver. You can also get bored with one vegetable if you eat it all the time. That's why his Cuisine for Cancer Prevention program works not with one or two promising vegetables, but with entire food families. "The underlying principle is that plants in the same botanical family have more similar compositions than plants from different families," he says.

Here's a quick rundown of some of the more interesting crucifers among broccoli's cousins.

KALE

Kale at a Glance
- Pigments: chlorophyll, lutein, beta-carotene
- Other phytochemicals: glucobrassicin (indole-3-carbinol), glucoraphanin (sulforaphane), sinigrin (allyl isothiocyanate), kaempferol, quercetin
- Serving size: one-half cup, cooked
- Vitamins and minerals per serving: A (96% of the Daily Value), C (45% DV), K (590% DV), manganese (13% DV), calcium (5% DV), potassium (4% DV), magnesium (3% DV), folate (2% DV)
- Fiber per serving: 5% DV
- ORAC score: 1,700

Benjamin Franklin was one of our wisest statesmen and Founding Fathers, so perhaps it's not surprising that he's credited with bringing the first kale seeds to the United States from Scotland. If any vegetable gives broccoli a run for its money, it's kale. It's almost as if kale were challenging broccoli with that old song, "Anything you can do, I can do better." It's got seven times more beta-carotene than broccoli and nearly 11 times more lutein. Ounce for ounce, it excels in vitamin K, with nearly 600 percent of the daily value. It delivers indole-3-carbinol and sulforaphane, plus a related compound called allyl isothiocyanate. And in antioxidant punch, kale is second only to watercress. OK, it falls short of broccoli on a few vitamins and minerals. But overall, the only reason why kale doesn't get as much attention as broccoli may be that doctors and dieticians think that trying to get people to eat it is a lost cause.

For those who are tempted to pass on kale, Melanie Polk, director of nutrition education at the American Institute for Cancer Research, notes that there are many ingenious ways to sneak chopped kale into soups and sauces without the family's noticing. "I once put finely chopped kale in lasagna and nobody knew it was there," she says. "I threw it into the food processor with some fresh carrots, then sautéed it lightly, and added the mixture to the pasta sauce." When Polk's daughter asked what the green flecks were, Polk claimed innocently that they were "probably oregano"—and got away with it. "I had the satisfaction of knowing I'd made a more nutritious dish," she says.

For those who are brave enough to eat kale undisguised, Dan Nadeau has included two of his own favorite recipes in the back of the book—Kale with Garlic, on page 268, and Sesame Kale, on page 269.

CABBAGE

Cabbage at a Glance
- Pigments: chlorophyll, lutein, beta-carotene
- Other phytochemicals: glucobrassicin (indole-3-carbinol), glucoraphanin (sulforaphane), butenyl-glucosinolate, glucoiberin, indoyl-methyl-glucosinolate, kaempferol, quercetin, chlorogenic acid
- Serving size: one-half cup, shredded
- Vitamins and minerals per serving: C (18% of the Daily Value), folate (4% DV), K (48% DV)
- Fiber per serving: 3% DV
- ORAC score: 298

There are certain staples, such as corn and potatoes, that have sustained populations throughout the ages. We don't often think of cabbage in this context, but it is another. In Chinese, the word for "cabbage" comes from the same root as the word for "vegetable," which gives a general idea of its importance in that culture. The Chinese consume many varieties of cabbage, including celery cabbage, flowering white cabbage, and bok choy—and they eat it almost every day. In northern Europe, too, cabbage was a staple for many centuries, providing an especially important winter food. That's because its tightly packed heads with their overlapping leaves grow well in cold weather, long after fragile heads of loosely-packed lettuce have succumbed to the frost. Until recently, cabbage was one of the few vegetables in Russia that was routinely available in stores euphemistically labeled "greengrocers."

If you're short on vegetables, cabbage isn't a bad one to have on hand. Like the other crucifers, cabbage delivers a solid supply of isothiocyanates. In a recent study in Shanghai, China, researchers followed 18,000 men over 11 years to see which of them would develop lung cancer—and found a protective effect from cabbage. "We didn't actually ask people how much cabbage they were eating," says Fung-Lung Chung of the American Health Foundation, "because people's recall is notoriously unreliable." Instead the researchers measured levels of isothiocyanates in the urine as a way of gauging consumption. In the end, the statistics said it all. Men without any detectable levels of isothiocyanates had a 36 percent greater chance of developing lung cancer. "We have known for a long time that cruciferous vegetables are protective," says Chung, "but this seems to confirm that the isothiocyanates are one reason why."

All the varieties of cabbage are good. Of course, the Color Code team likes colorful purple cabbage even better than the standard variety, which is white on the inside. Purple cabbage has anthocyanins and nearly twice the vitamin C of green-white cabbage. Unfortunately, it has only half the folate.

WATERCRESS

Watercress at a Glance
- Pigments: chlorophyll, lutein, beta-carotene
- Other phytochemicals: gluconasturtiin (phenethyl isothio-

cyanate), glucoraphanin (sulforaphane), glucobrassicin (indole-3-carbinol)
- Serving size: 10 sprigs
- Vitamins and minerals per serving: A (16% of the Daily Value), C (15% DV), calcium (2% DV)
- Fiber per serving: 2% DV
- ORAC score: 2,200 (measured by Brunswick Labs)

Watercress is perhaps the most noble of the crucifers—and if anyone needs any proof of that, consider that King Louis IX of France awarded one French town a coat of arms emblazoned with three bunches of watercress! The king is said to have been impressed by the cool, refreshing qualities of the watercress he was served there on a hot day. Over the centuries, watercress has impressed plenty of other people, too. The ancient Greeks and Romans thought it could confer strength, courage, character, and even wit. In the Middle Ages, it was believed to prevent baldness, cure toothaches, and purify the blood and skin. We won't vouch for any of these. But watercress does boast a healthy amount of vitamins A and C, for a bare minimum of calories. A serving of 10 sprigs will cost you just five calories.

Watercress has been called the salad green that bites back—and by now it should come as no surprise that the bitter taste in watercress is due to its isothiocyanates. Watercress has an unusual one, called *phenethyl isothiocyanate*—or PEITC, for short. You can find PEITC in bok choy, turnips, and turnip greens, too, but by far the best source is watercress. It turns out that PEITC is particularly good at combating a series of cancer-causing nitrosamines in tobacco smoke. That means that it not only appears to fight lung cancer, but also esophageal tumors that are caused by these tobacco-specific carcinogens. In one study, Stephen Hecht, a biochemist at the University of Minnesota Cancer Center in Minneapolis, gave a potent nitrosamine called NNK to a group of rats. More than 70 percent of them developed lung tumors. A second group of rats received both cancer-inducing NNK and protective PEITC. The results? Fewer than 10 percent of the PEITC-protected rats developed tumors.

Hecht took his work one step further and tried a small study with 11 smokers. He fed them two ounces of watercress three times a day for three days. Then he measured the chemicals in their urine. On the watercress diet, the smokers excreted higher quantities of NNK detoxification products than when they ate no watercress. Apparently NNK was being ushered out of the body instead of lingering to cause ill effects. Of course, this doesn't prove that PEITC would ultimately prevent lung cancer in these smokers, as it did in rats. Few people eat anywhere near enough watercress, and there are other carcinogens in tobacco smoke that PEITC does not work against. But as a component of a healthy cancer-prevention diet, it is at least promising.

BRUSSELS SPROUTS

Brussels Sprouts at a Glance
- Pigments: chlorophyll, lutein, beta-carotene
- Other phytochemicals: glucobrassicin (indole-3-carbinol), *p*-coumaric acid, D-glucaric acid, caffeic acid, ferulic acid, alpha-lipoic acid
- Serving size: four sprouts
- Vitamins and minerals per serving: A (8% of the Daily Value), C (120% DV), K (243% DV), calcium (2% DV)
- Fiber per serving: 12% DV
- ORAC score: 980

There are no prizes for guessing where Brussels sprouts originated. Although some early versions may have been cultivated in ancient Rome, the Brussels sprouts that we know today were first grown in large quantities in France and Belgium, particularly around the Belgian capital. As such, these crucifers are thought to be one of only two common vegetables that originated in northern Europe. (The other is kohlrabi.)

Despite the name, Brussels sprouts aren't really sprouts at all. They're small cabbages. The difference is that standard cabbage grows in a single head atop a very short stalk. By contrast, Brussels sprouts have a long stem growing out of the ground, with many tiny cabbage heads, or sprouts, along the stem. Each of those tiny cabbage heads comes with the health benefits of its larger sibling. For example, Alan Kristal at the Fred Hutchinson Cancer Research Center found in one study that men who ate four servings of vegetables a day had a 35 percent lower risk of prostate cancer than those who ate just two. In particular, he found that cruciferous vegetables—broccoli, cabbage, sauerkraut, Brussels sprouts, and cauliflower—reduced the risk by 41 percent in those who ate three servings a week as opposed to one a week. Cruciferous vegetables, he noted, reduced prostate-cancer risk even more than lycopene-rich tomatoes!

Kiwifruit
Kiwifruit is practically synonymous with New Zealand. It was named for New Zealand's national bird, the kiwi. New Zealanders in general and the national soccer team in particular are called Kiwis, too. So you would be excused for thinking that kiwifruit is native to this nation. It isn't. These small fuzzy fruits originally came from the Yangtze River Valley in China, where they were known as *yangtao*. It wasn't until the early 1900s that a visiting New Zealander took some "Chinese gooseberry" seeds home, and a national industry grew out of it. When an export market developed, proud New Zealanders rechristened the fruits "kiwis," and so they have been named ever since.

No matter what you call them, these fruits are exceptional sources of vitamins and minerals. One serving of two medium kiwis gives you nearly twice the vitamin C of an orange. Ounce for ounce, kiwis are higher in vitamin C than any other fruit except guava. They also pack plenty of potassium, magnesium, and lutein. And they're the only fruit other than the avocado that's green when fully mature! Here's a look at the good stuff in kiwis:

- Pigments: lutein, beta-carotene, beta-cryptoxanthin, zeaxanthin, chlorophyll
- Other phytochemicals: tannins
- Serving size: 2 medium kiwis
- Vitamins and minerals per serving: A (2% of the Daily Value), C (240% DV), folate (17% DV), E (10% DV), B_6 (5% DV), potassium (10% DV), calcium (6% DV)

- Fiber per serving: 16% DV
- ORAC score: 602

By the way, if the fuzzy brown exterior of kiwis stops you from buying them, there's a miniature fuzz-less kiwi that's recently begun appearing in specialty stores. The miniatures grow in clusters like grapes on a trellis and are even higher in nutrients than regular kiwis, with one big plus: You can easily eat the skin.

GREEN TEA

Tea at a Glance
- Pigments: theaflavins, thearubigens (black tea); chlorophyll (green tea)
- Other phytochemicals: epicatechin, epigallocatechin, epigallocatechin gallate (green tea); gallic acid, theogallin, caffeine, theobromine, quercetin, rutin, apigenin, chlorogenic acid, cinnamic acid, kaempferol, myricetin
- Vitamins and minerals: traces of riboflavin, niacin, potassium, calcium, magnesium
- ORAC score: 831

As legend has it, the Chinese emperor Shen Nung was relaxing in the shade of a tree one day in 2737 B.C., while his servant boiled some drinking water. A breeze came up, and a few leaves from the tree—a wild tea tree—fluttered into the pot. The emperor decided to drink the water anyway and was delighted with the result. Over the centuries, tea became enshrined in Chinese life. The Tang Dynasty scholar Luk Yu praised it in his classic *Book of Tea* as "the sweetest dew from Heaven." Buddhist monks from Japan apparently agreed. Their reverence for tea spawned the elaborate Japanese tea ceremony.

In the 17th century, the Dutch and English began importing tea from China. In the Netherlands, the reception was somewhat cold at first. Doctors were the only people who initially expressed interest in the new "hay water." In England, however, tea rapidly gained favor. On June 28, 1667, the great diarist Samuel Pepys recorded that he "arrived home and found my wife making a tea, a drink Mr. Pelling [the apothecary] tells her is good for her cold." The British East India company soon began advertising tea as a cure for just about everything, including apoplexy, colic, consumption, drowsiness, epilepsy, gallstones, migraine, paralysis, and vertigo. Belief in these powers gradually faded, but the popularity of tea did not. In the early 1800s, Anna, wife of the seventh duke of Bedford, even elevated it a notch by calling for tea and light refreshments in the afternoon to stave off a "sinking feeling." Ever since then, the custom of afternoon tea has been as English as Buckingham Palace.

One Leaf, Three Teas

Today we know that tea truly is a healthy drink. It does not cure apoplexy and vertigo, but evidence is mounting that it can help prevent heart disease, stroke, cancer, and a variety of other ailments. That's because it is an exceptionally rich source of polyphenolic compounds. To date, most of the health research has focused on green tea, but black tea appears to be equally protective. That's hardly surprising. The two teas come from the same plant, *Camellia sinensis*. The difference is in the processing. In short, black tea has been allowed to oxidize and green tea has not.

When you chop fresh tea leaves, this activates an enzyme called polyphenol oxidase. As the name implies, the enzyme causes the rapid oxidation of polyphenols in the leaves. If they are allowed to sit for the next 90 minutes or so, about 80 percent of the polyphenols will oxidize. The result: black tea. If, however, the leaves are steamed first, heat deactivates the enzyme, and the polyphenols remain unoxidized. The result: green tea. Oolong is the compromise—the same tea leaves partially oxidized.

How does oxidation affect the health-conferring components of tea? The most abundant and powerful cancer fighter in green tea is a flavonoid called—ready for this?—*epigallocatechin gallate*, or EGCG. Lab studies indicate that it's one of the most potent antioxidants we consume. But during the oxidation of tea, EGCG and related catechins are converted into compounds called theaflavins and thearubigens. That means that the major antioxidant and cancer fighter in green tea is not present in black tea to any great extent. But here's the interesting thing. Evidence is emerging that the polyphenols in black tea are just as effective as those in green tea. "The only reason that green tea has a better reputation is that Chinese and Japanese scientists started studying tea many years before Western researchers did," says John Weisburger, a senior member of the American Health Foundation. "Naturally they studied green tea, since that's what they drink."

Sip a Cuppa for Your Heart

Certainly evidence is emerging that both teas fight cardiovascular disease, including strokes. In one Japanese study, 5,910 women were followed for four years to see if green tea could decrease their stroke rates. It did. Those who drank five or more cups a day suffered half as many strokes as those who sipped less. But black tea appears equally effective. In the famous Zutphen Elderly Study in the Netherlands, three quercetin-rich foods protected Dutch men against strokes—apples, onions, and tea. Of these, tea— black tea—was the most effective by far. Over the 15 years of the study, men who drank five cups a day reduced their risk of stroke by a dramatic 70 percent. Similarly, the Rotterdam Study found that Dutch men and women who sipped four cups a day cut their risks of severe atherosclerosis by 70 percent. Even the one-to-two-cup crowd lowered their risks of severe atherosclerosis by an impressive 46 percent. The question is why.

There are several possible explanations. As you already know, oxidation plays a role in the development of heart disease. When "bad" cholesterol is oxidized, it can set off a downward spiral leading to hardening of the arteries, heart attack, and stroke. The polyphenols in tea may help prevent that, with their antioxidant strength. In addition, unspecified components of tea appear to reduce the amount of cholesterol in the blood, apparently by interfering with the absorption of dietary fats and cholesterol.

Tea does something else, too. According to Dr. Joseph Vita of Boston University School of Medicine, it improves the function of the vascular endothelium, which lines artery walls. This layer of cells controls the dilation and constriction of blood vessels, in accordance with the varying needs of the body for blood-borne oxygen and nutrients. When it is healthy, blood vessels are not as likely to thicken or form plaques. Endothelial function is often measured by the ability of arteries to dilate. This is what Vita measured in a new study involving 50 patients with coronary artery disease. Participants drank four cups of tea every day for a month, then switched and drank water instead for a month. In a normal person, arteries can expand by up to 13 percent. But in Vita's patients, they dilated only 6 percent at the outset of the trial. After a month of tea, however, there was a marked improvement. Blood vessels could widen 9 to 10 percent. Water made no difference. "Our study doesn't prove that tea prevents heart disease, but it helps explain why it might reduce the risk," says Vita. He himself has started drinking tea more often, "now that I know it's good for my arteries."

Cancer Control

Tea also appears to be good at fighting cancer, especially malignancies of the gastrointestinal tract. In Japan the people of Shizuoka Prefecture, a tea-producing region, have particularly low levels of stomach, esophageal, and liver cancers. In Shanghai, China, those who drink the most green tea have the lowest rates of esophageal cancer. The evidence is not entirely consistent. There are also some large studies that show no effects from tea consumption. But that may be because tea is prepared in so many different ways worldwide—from hot to iced, from sweetened to salted and buttered (in Tibet). Preparation can make a huge difference. In the United States, researchers at the Arizona Cancer Center in Tucson recently found no correlation between skin cancer rates and the consumption of tea in general—but a 37 percent decrease in skin cancer among those who drank two cups of *hot black* tea a day. "Bottled teas and ice teas are too diluted to do much good," says Dr. Iman Hakim, the preventive oncologist who led the study. "Boiling the water will extract more of the polyphenols, and so will leaving the bag in for several minutes."

Through laboratory research, scientists have found that tea apparently intervenes in multiple ways to stop tumor formation and development.

Right up front, it helps protect against cancer-causing assaults by zapping free radicals and boosting detoxification enzymes.

If cells do develop mutations, tea can also help prevent them from progressing to cancer. Allan Conney of Rutgers University gave hairless mice either green tea or water to drink for two weeks. He then exposed the mice to a single dose of ultraviolet light, enough to cause mutations in skin cells. In self-defense, a protective "tumor-suppressor" gene in the mice swung into action. This so-called *p53* gene produces chemicals that cause abnormal cells to self-destruct. "The abnormal cells are eliminated from the animal and do not go on to become cancerous," says Conney. In both sets of mice, the *p53* mechanism rushed to the rescue. In the tea group, however, the protective effect was doubled.

But what if tumors have already formed? Can tea help squelch those, too? The answer appears to be yes—at least in lab animals. Conney took mice with skin tumors and divided them into two groups. One group received black tea as their sole source of drinking fluid for 11 weeks. The control group received water. At the end, Conney found that the tumors in the tea-drinking mice were 70 percent smaller than those in the non–tea-drinkers. Later examination showed that tea was inhibiting DNA synthesis—and without DNA synthesis, you can't get the proliferation of new cells. Tumor cells in the tea drinkers were also more likely to self-destruct through apoptosis.

Tea may possibly even help at the final, deadly stage of cancer—metastasis, where tumor cells spread to other tissues of the body. Japanese researchers have shown that EGCG can slow the metastasis of melanoma cells in mice, although much more work needs to be done to confirm this finding.

The Healthiest Cup of Tea

Tea is an ideal food for cancer prevention, because it's low in cost and people actually like it. Next to water, it is the most commonly consumed beverage worldwide. But as we've said, the method of preparation can greatly affect its potency.

The best is brewed tea, either black or green. Let it steep for at least three minutes to extract the greatest number of healthful phytochemicals. (The more of these that you can draw from the tea leaves into the water, the more colorful the tea will be—and the more benefits it will deliver.) Just remember to let the tea cool a little before drinking it. Some studies have indicated that consumption of scalding tea over a period of many years will only irritate the throat and actually increase the risk for esophageal cancer.

If you want maximum protection, steer clear of fancy bottled drinks and iced teas. A *Consumer Reports* study found that instant teas had significantly less antioxidant activity than fresh-brewed teas. Bottled teas had still less. Of course, the added sugar doesn't contribute any protective benefits.

If you don't tolerate caffeine well, decaffeinated teas are fine, but you'll lose some of their disease-fighting power. In Allan Conney's studies at Rutgers University, he found that a substantial portion of the cancer-fighting potential came from the caffeine.

For those avoiding caffeine, herbal teas also have many wonderful phytochemicals and antioxidants. Chamomile tea, for one, has been studied for its anti-inflammatory and antibacterial properties; chamomile has been used to relieve indigestion, ulcers, and cramps. But herbal teas are not true teas, so don't expect them to deliver precisely the same benefits as either green or black tea.

The "Hot" New Diet Drink

As an added benefit, it is just possible that tea could help you lose weight—not lots of weight, but maybe a pound or two. A series of Swiss studies found that tea can give your metabolism a lift. Of course, one reason would be the caffeine, which serves as a stimulant. But these studies found that the effect was larger than the caffeine alone could deliver. The scientists suspect that the polyphenols and caffeine join forces to unblock the fat-burning process at different control points.

HERBS

Are you going to Scarborough Fair?
Parsley, sage, rosemary and thyme.
Remember me to one who lives there.
She once was a true love of mine.
              —old English song

"There's rosemary, that's for remembrance," says Ophelia in *Hamlet*. For centuries, in fact, rosemary has been associated with memory. In ancient Greece, students were said to have braided rosemary into their hair to help them on exams. In Virginia's historic Jamestown Settlement today, costumed interpreters wear sprigs of rosemary tucked into their hair, as the early settlers would have done to remind themselves of home and of loved ones left behind.

If rosemary does aid memory, that may well be because of its antioxidant effect. In studies at Rutgers University, Chi-Tang Ho found that sage, rosemary, and thyme were all strong antioxidants. You may not eat large amounts of any of these. But researchers are now realizing that there's value in them anyway. "For years, we added herbs to foods to make them taste better," says nutritionist Melanie Polk. "Now we know that by adding herbs and spices, you're adding protective phytochemicals, just as if you were eating fruits and vegetables." And by enhancing flavor, herbs and spices allow you to reduce the salt you would add, too.

Of all the dietary herbs, rosemary may have the most research behind it. Studies have shown that the fresh leaves contain one particularly interesting antioxidant—a terpenoid called *carnosic acid*. "The beauty of carnosic acid is that a single molecule can grab a lot of free radicals," says Carolyn Fisher, an organic chemist at McCormick & Co. Carnosic acid quenches two free radicals, then rearranges itself to form another compound, *carnosol,* which grabs two more free radicals before rearranging itself yet again to swipe at two more. In studies at Rutgers University, Allan Conney has found that rosemary extracts inhibit skin cancer in mice very effectively. No doubt that's due in part to carnosic acid's antioxidant strength. But rosemary functions in other ways, too. It also promotes detoxification, prevents carcinogens from binding to DNA, and stems the chronic inflammation that contributes to cancer development. There are no studies in human populations, but every indication is that rosemary should promote health.

So should related herbs, such as sage and thyme. Thyme contains a number of familiar cancer-fighting polyphenols, such as *p*-coumaric acid and chlorogenic acid. It also contains potent terpenoids, such as the antimicrobials *carvacrol* and *thymol*. Both are capable of killing oral bacteria and certain food-borne pathogens. Thyme also contains cancer-fighting *geraniol,* another terpenoid. Of course, you don't get a lot of any of these compounds in a sprinkling of herbs. But many scientists now believe that small doses of a great many phytochemicals may be just as effective as large doses of a single compound.

All in the Family

Rosemary, sage, and thyme are all members of the extended mint family. Not surprisingly, mint itself is no slouch. "In China, when you get a cold, your mother makes you drink tea with lemon and mint," says Zhi Yuan Wang, a cancer research scientist who is working with the American Health Foundation. "We used to regard it as folk medicine. Now we know that mint contains a lot of terpenes that act as antioxidants and detoxifiers." Of course, mint contains sinus-clearing *menthol,* a terpenoid that is closely related in structure to limonene. It also contains perillyl alcohol, which is emerging as a potent cancer fighter. Lab studies show that perillyl alcohol both slows the division of cancer cells and increases their rate of programmed cell death. In rats, it battles mammary tumors. In hamsters, it shrinks pancreatic tumors and even makes some of these cancers completely disappear. The results are so promising that early trials for perillyl alcohol have begun in humans, but with doses far larger than you would find in foods.

The list of beneficial phytochemicals in herbs goes on and on. If it's oregano you sprinkle on your pizza, you'll be getting a good dose of farnesol. In studies with its derivative, *farnesyl anthranilate,* Charles Elson of the University of Wisconsin has found that minute amounts in the diet can block the growth of a certain type of fast-growing skin tumor in mice. Japanese studies have also shown oregano to be a potent antioxidant. Lemon grass contains geraniol, a citrusy terpenoid that also appears to fight cancer. Basil also contains geraniol, in addition to eugenol, kaempferol, myrcene, quercetin, rutin, caffeic acid, and thymol. In fact, it's hard to find an herb or spice that isn't loaded with beneficial, aromatic compounds.

Fresh herbs are, naturally, the best. They're the most flavorful, and they deliver the most phytochemicals. But dried herbs will do, if the bottles or jars haven't lingered too long on your kitchen shelf. You can dry your own herbs in the microwave. Start by separating the leaves from the stems. Then spread the leaves in a thin layer on a double thickness of paper towels. A total of four to six minutes in the microwave will do the job. It's a good idea to pause the microwave a couple times to shift the leaves for more even drying. The herbs will be very brittle when done. Store them in airtight containers.

BLUE-PURPLE

5

"I believe a leaf of grass is no less than the journey work of
the stars, . . .
And the running blackberry would adorn the parlors of
heaven."
—Walt Whitman, "Song of Myself" from *Leaves of Grass*

IMAGINE A DELICATE TROPICAL BREEZE, the sound of waves lapping the shore, and pure white sand caressing your feet. You gaze at a soft horizon, where the azure blue of the sky meets the majestic blue of the sea. Without a care in the world, you bask in the relaxing blueness of it all.

More than any other color, blue means stress reduction. Just as an idyllic week on a secluded beach relaxes the mind, blue and purple foods relieve the body from the oxidative stress of free radicals. In the ORAC tests at Tufts, blue foods quenched more free radicals than any other foods. Blueberries and blackberries were clear winners among fresh fruits; prunes and raisins, among dried fruits. That's at least in part because they deliver such intense doses of protective anthocyanin pigments. So go ahead and relax—enjoy a cup of blueberries.

BLUEBERRIES

Blueberries at a Glance
- Pigments: anthocyanins (multiple forms of cyanidin, delphinidin, malvidin, peonidin, and petunidin), beta-carotene

- Other phytochemicals: chlorogenic acid, kaempferol, myricetin, *p*-coumaric acid, quercetin, ferulic acid, condensed tannins (proanthocyanidins), fructooligosaccharides, resveratrol
- Serving size: one cup
- Vitamins and minerals per serving: C (32% of the Daily Value), A (6% DV), E (4% DV), potassium (4% DV), folate (4% DV), iron (2% DV), zinc (2% DV)
- Fiber per serving: 8% DV
- ORAC score: 2,400

We're almost at the end of our palette of colorful foods. But don't close the book now. In many ways, we've saved the most exciting foods for last, including one that shows exceptional promise—the blueberry. This blue jewel is the Lady Di, the Princess Grace, the Sophia Loren of fruits. It is a sophisticated, complicated member of the *Vaccinium* genus of berries, not to mention a virtual storehouse of antioxidant and anti-inflammatory compounds. Unfortunately, until very recently this wonderful fruit was relegated to bit parts in the American diet. But Jim Joseph's research at Tufts University is helping to change that. Jim has made headline news across the country by showing that blueberries confer true "anti-aging" benefits. They don't "merely" help prevent declines in old age. They actually appear to *reverse* some aspects of brain aging, at least in animal studies. If all this research is ultimately borne out in human trials, this humble berry could turn out to be one of the most important additions to a healthy diet. It's also one of the few ways to round out your color palette with a blue food for the day.

The Great Spirit and the Star Berry

The blueberry is a true-blue American, a fruit that originated in North America. For centuries before the arrival of Europeans on these shores, Native Americans treasured these "star" berries—so called because the blossom end of each blueberry forms a five-pointed star. They used blueberries to flavor soups and stews, and to form the base of a delicious honeyed pudding. They even pounded them into dried meat cakes, which kept for up to two years, thanks to the berries' antioxidant strength. One of the first meals that the explorers Lewis and Clark shared with Native Americans was venison prepared in this way. Native Americans also valued blueberries for their medicinal properties. They brewed the berries, roots, and leaves into teas and syrups to treat diarrhea and to ease childbirth. Blueberries were so important to survival that the Native Americans believed the Great Spirit had sent the star berries to preserve them in times of scarcity.

Despite these many uses, it was not until the early 1900s that anyone thought of cultivating blueberries. Elizabeth White, whose family harvested cranberries in the New Jersey Pine Barrens, was looking for another crop to supplement the family income. Blueberries seemed to fit the bill. White hired people to scour the land for the wild bushes with the largest fruits, then worked with the New Jersey Department of Agriculture to develop cultivated berries from these plants, each of which was named for the individuals who found it. This practice occasionally produced unappetizing names, as when Rube Leek collected a promising berry. No one would want a blueberry that was named "Leek"—and "Rube" just didn't send the right message. It became the "Rubel" instead. Even though customers today are rarely aware of the variety names, the Rubel blueberry is still grown.

Antioxidant Champions

Nutritionists have long regarded blueberries as nutritional weaklings, but that opinion is rapidly changing. True, blueberries do not contain scurvy-banishing amounts of vitamin C or heroic quantities of vitamin A. But they are the undisputed antioxidant champions among fresh fruits and vegetables. In the ORAC tests at Tufts, blueberries beat out about 50 other fresh fruits and vegetables—in other words, every fresh food that the Tufts team tested. In 1998, *Eating Well* magazine named blueberries Fruit of the Year. Health writers around the country soon followed up with accolades of their own. "If you add one food to your diet this year, make it blueberries," wrote dietician Holly McCord in *Prevention* magazine.

The awesome antioxidant power of blueberries comes from

QUICK 'N' EASY

Blueberries are so good eaten fresh, there's really no need for special recipes. But creative chefs have nevertheless devised plenty of novel ways to use blueberries in foods. If you visit Bar Harbor, Maine, during wild blueberry season, you'll find a wealth of blueberry-based treats, from salad dressings to sorbets. One of our favorite recipes, from chef William Sellner Jr. at Michelle's Fine Dining in Bar Harbor, is for a fabulous wild blueberry soup that's simple to make, too. You'll find the recipe on page 232.

Another super simple and highly nutritious treat is blueberry-banana smoothies. Dan Nadeau makes his from wild Maine blueberries, which he gets fresh or frozen from the store, but cultivated berries taste just as good. Dan swears he feels stress slipping away with every sip of this delicious drink. His recipe appears on page 290.

two main sources, according to food chemist Wilhelmina Kalt of Agriculture and Agri-Food Canada, the Canadian equivalent of the USDA. One is chlorogenic acid, which is among the cancer fighters in tomatoes and bell peppers. Chlorogenic acid is found in large quantities in blueberries. The other source of antioxidant power is the anthocyanin pigments that give blueberries their intense color. "In some fruits, you'll find three, four, perhaps five types of anthocyanins," says Kalt. "Wild blueberries can have as many as twenty-five or thirty." It's not that the individual anthocyanins in blueberries are stronger than those in other fruits. It's that blueberries have so darn many types and in such large concentrations. That means that the antioxidant power in blueberries comes literally "out of the blue."

Blueberries also appear to contain potent anti-inflammatories, including the pigment cyanidin, which contributes to the arthritis-relieving effects of tart cherries.

The Virtues of the "Brain Berry"

All these antioxidants and anti-inflammatories may make blueberries one of the best foods for protecting the brain as we age. Think of it this way. Just as the Earth is protected from meteors by its atmosphere, an "atmosphere" of antioxidants and anti-inflammatories protects our brains from free-radical hits. Without the earth's protective atmosphere, our planet would soon be barren and pockmarked, like the surface of the moon. Similarly our brains, without any protection against free radicals and inflammatories, would deteriorate until they were moonlike and barren in their functioning. Fortunately, we have safeguards in the form of antioxidants and anti-inflammatories—and some of the best come from blueberries. They appear to be so protective of the brain that plant physiologist Mary Ann Lila Smith at the University of Illinois has dubbed the blueberry the "brain berry."

The most dramatic evidence of the brain berry's powers has come from Jim Joseph's lab at Tufts. Assuming that oxidative stress and inflammation contribute to brain aging, Jim wanted to see if blueberries could reduce or even reverse some of the negative effects. To test his idea, he used aging rats. In human terms, these animals were between 65 and 70 years old. Not surprisingly, at the outset of the study they were already showing declines in memory, motor coordination, and balance. Jim and his colleague Barbara Shukitt-Hale fed the animals either a control diet or a diet supplemented with 1 to 2 percent blueberries, strawberries, or spinach that had been made into a freeze-dried powder. (In human terms, this is the equivalent of a half to a whole cup of blueberries, a pint of strawberries, or a large spinach salad.)

After two months on this diet, the animals were given a test called the Morris water maze, which measures memory. In this test, the animals paddle around a deep pool until they find a submerged platform where they can rest. The question is how quickly they can find it the next time. They can't see the platform itself, because it is under water, but objects around the side of the pool serve as visual cues—including a soda bottle, a broom, and a poster of wild Maine blueberries. As it turns out, the rats on the blueberry, strawberry, and spinach diets were able to remember the location of the platform better and were able to find it more quickly than control rats on the standard diet.

What was really striking, however, was the rats' performance in a series of athletic tests that Jim dubbed the Rat Olympics. The blueberry-fed rats not only outperformed the other animals, but also showed actual improvements in coordination and balance. They were able to stay atop a narrow beam for 11 seconds—versus just 6 seconds for those on the standard diet. On the "lumberjack test," the blueberry-fed rats kept their balance on a spinning rod for 9 seconds—more than twice as long as the control group on the standard diet. What's more, in a related study at the Denver Veterans Affairs Medical Center, Jim's colleague Paula Bickford found that blueberry- and spinach-fed rats quickly made their way across a narrow, ladder-like runway in which some of the pegs had been removed. Rats on the standard diet took much longer to figure it out. Clearly, blueberries help the brain. But how?

Additional testing has revealed three possible ways. First, the blueberry-fed rats in Jim's experiments actually developed new brain cells at a greater rate than the others. Until recently, it was considered impossible to grow new neurons at all. Scientists thought that an animal—or a person, for that matter—was born with all the brain cells he or she would ever have. But in recent years, research at Princeton University and the Salk Institute has shown that both animals and humans can and do grow new neurons. Jim's rats did, too—but the blueberry-fed group developed more than the others.

Second, brain cells in the blueberry-fed rats actually seemed to communicate better. As we age, the opposite usually happens. Receptors on the surface of these cells grow less responsive to chemical messengers. When brain cells don't respond well to signals, that translates into declines in balance and coordination, for starters. But two types of receptors actually became more sensitive in the blueberry group.

Finally, as we age, our brains start having trouble cleaning up damaged proteins. These proteins can clutter the brain, interfering with neuronal communications. The blueberry-fed rats, however, had fewer damaged proteins in their brains.

None of these improvements made the rats young again. They

still lagged far behind "teenage" rats. But turning back the clock even a little is better than turning it forward. If similar improvements are possible in humans, these gains may be enough to keep the elderly independent longer and improve their quality of life.

Sweetening the Pot

Those are some pretty good reasons for including these little blue jewels in your diet, but let's "sweeten" the pot just a bit more. Blueberries, it turns out, may also hinder the onset of Alzheimer's disease.

Together with David Morgan and Gary Arendash at the University of South Florida, Jim ran some tests on genetically-altered mice. Unlike normal mice, these rodents develop high levels of a substance called amyloid beta, which forms insoluble plaques in their brains. These plaques are one of the two biological hallmarks of Alzheimer's disease in humans.

As soon as the mice could be weaned, they were divided into two groups. One group received a standard diet until the age of 12 months (which is middle-aged in these mice). The other group was given a blueberry-supplemented regimen. Both groups developed amyloid plaques, but there was a crucial difference: Despite the presence of plaques, the blueberry-fed group continued to perform well on a test of cognitive function called the Y maze. A normal, curious mouse will explore all three arms of the Y-shaped structure, moving from one arm to the next repeatedly during a five-minute interval. So will a genetically-altered mouse whose diet includes the blueberry supplement. But an "Alzheimer-like" mouse on the standard diet will tend to go back to the same arm over and over. This mouse demonstrates less curiosity and capacity for engaging with the environment, just like a person with Alzheimer's disease. Why do the blueberry-fed mice do so much better? According to Jim, the color-fed group has higher levels of enzymes and proteins that aid normal communications among brain cells.

Of course, this doesn't guarantee that blueberries will prevent or delay the onset of Alzheimer's disease in people. It's just an early indication that they might be helpful. Jim also cautions, "The mice were given blueberries before they developed any pathology. Once you've got the disease, it may be too late." So why wait? Start eating blueberries now.

Heavy-Particle Radiation

Jim has conducted one more set of very interesting experiments. Working with Barbara Shukitt-Hale in his lab and Bernard Rabin from the University of Maryland, Baltimore County, he has subjected rats to heavy-particle radiation—the same type of radiation that astronauts are exposed to in space. Of course, most of us will never go into space. But that doesn't mean this experiment is irrelevant for us. This type of radiation also causes accelerated aging— and all of us will age. In this set of tests, Jim found two very interesting things. A blueberry- or strawberry-supplemented diet not only blocked some of the effects of radiation on the brain, but it also prevented radiation sickness. Jim is still collecting data, but he says, "If you can expose a rat to radiation and the animal shows no ill effects, that's pretty amazing."

Bilberry Jam: The Secret Weapon?

During World War II, the Allies had a secret weapon—the bilberry, or the European version of the blueberry. Before night missions, British Royal Air Force pilots ate bilberry jam to improve their night vision. Does it really help? A series of European studies with air-traffic controllers, pilots, and truck drivers in the 1960s confirmed that bilberry extracts containing anthocyanins and beta-carotene really did work—probably because they increased the regeneration rate of "visual purple," the purple pigment in the retina that allows us to see in dim light. Bilberry extracts also appear to strengthen the capillaries in the eyes, improving circulation to the retina.

Do American blueberries work as well as European bilberries? No one has done that research. But we should point out that bilberries, unlike blueberries, have pigments in their flesh as well as in their skins and are therefore probably even more potent. You can't go wrong with that much blue!

Pie in the Sky

Does all this good news about blueberries mean that you can obtain eternal youth by eating blueberry pie? Well, no. "Cooking can be quite damaging to the antioxidant capacity of blueberries," says food chemist Wilhelmina Kalt. "The anthocyanins are susceptible to heat damage." If you start with canned pie filling, which has been heated once, the anthocyanin levels are already lower than in raw fruit. Once you bake the pie, they're lower still. "The message is, raw is better than cooked," says Kalt. Think of it as one more reason to drink blueberry smoothies.

BLACKBERRIES

Blackberries at a Glance
- Pigments: anthocyanins (various forms of cyanidin)
- Other phytochemicals: chlorogenic acid, ellagic acid, catechins, ferulic acid, gallic acid, kaempferol, quercetin
- Serving size: one cup
- Vitamins and minerals per serving: C (50% of the Daily Value), folate (12% DV), E (6% DV), manganese (93% DV), potassium (8% DV), magnesium (7% DV), calcium (5% DV), iron (5% DV)
- Fiber per serving: 30% DV
- ORAC score: 2,036

If you ever treat yourself to a drive along the back roads of Oregon's Willamette Valley, you will find a profusion of brambles growing along the roadside. In late summer, these sprawling vines are laden with juicy, black gems that make mouthwatering treats. "When I first moved here, I was amazed that you could get these incredible berries for free, all over the place," says Cat McKenzie of the Oregon Raspberry and Blackberry Commission. Oregon's temperate climate is perfect for blackberries, both wild and cultivated. The winters are mild, and the summers are filled with warm days and cool nights. Those low evening temperatures slow the ripening process, allowing the berries to remain longer on the vine—and the longer they stay on the vine, the more rich and complex the flavor becomes.

Flavor is one good reason to eat blackberries, but it's not the only one. There's also a burgeoning list of health reasons. "In the past, we would have said the main reason to eat blackberries was vitamin C," says Ronald Wrolstad, distinguished professor of food science and technology at Oregon State University. "Then we learned about potassium." Next came folate and a heaping helping of fiber, including cholesterol-lowering pectin. And to top it off, says Wrolstad, "Today, we're learning that blackberries are rich in polyphenolics, including anthocyanin pigments."

Blackberries are loaded with these pigments, as a quick glance at the berries will readily tell you. That's no doubt one reason why they're such potent antioxidants. They placed right after blueberries in the ORAC tests at Tufts, with an outstanding score of 2,036. In addition, blackberries are full of disease-proofing phytochemicals. Perhaps most notably, the fiber-rich seeds contain high levels of ellagic acid. In lab studies, ellagic acid has been shown to battle cancer on several fronts at once—decreasing the activity of the phase 1 enzymes that create certain carcinogens, boosting detoxifying phase 2 enzymes, and also encouraging apoptosis (programmed cell death) in diseased cells. True, blackberries don't turn up in epidemiological studies as protective against heart disease or cancer, but that could be because most people simply don't eat enough of them.

As with most fruits, blackberries come in several varieties. Consumers are not often aware of specific varietal names, but one that may have come to your attention is the Marion blackberry, or Marionberry. (As Jim Joseph notes, that's no relation to the former mayor of Washington, D.C.) Named for Marion County, Oregon, where it was bred, the Marionberry can be found fresh only in Oregon, but it is shipped frozen across the country. "Marionberries have an incredible, more complex flavor than regular blackberries," says Jan Schroeder, executive director of the Oregon Raspberry and Blackberry Commission. "We call them the cabernet sauvignon of blackberries. When you bake a Marionberry pie, you'll find neighbors knocking on your door."

There are also a number of blackberry-raspberry hybrids that you may know by name. Loganberries are one. They are named for Judge J. H. Logan, who accidentally bred them when he planted a raspberry bush too close to his blackberries. Boysenberries—named for horticulturalist Rudolph Boysen—are a cross between blackberries and loganberries. All are good—and good for you, too!

Q UICK 'N' EASY
    Trendy restaurants around the country have recently
discovered Marionberries. Stacie Pierce, the pastry chef at
March restaurant in New York, has concocted numerous
desserts that draw raves, including this one for Marionberries in a blood orange sauce. It's so easy to make that you
don't need a formal recipe. Pierce mixes a little sugar with
a dash of cinnamon and some flecks of fresh vanilla, and
she sprinkles the mixture on some carefully thawed
berries. She then squeezes a couple blood oranges over the
berries, adds a dusting of orange zest on top, and garnishes
it with a cinnamon stick. It's fabulous and elegant, too!

Fresh, Frozen, or Canned?

When Dan Nadeau talks to his patients about eating fruits and
vegetables, they often ask if it's OK to eat frozen or canned foods
instead of fresh, especially during the winter. The answer is a qual-
ified yes.

Fresh produce is still the ideal—especially if it's fresh out of the
garden or grown locally. That way, picked at the peak of ripeness,
it has the highest levels of phytonutrients. But let's face it, we're
not generally buying garden-fresh foods at the grocery store. The
produce in supermarkets has usually spent a couple days in transit
and several more days on store shelves. Although it's kept cool to
preserve it, you inevitably lose a small fraction of nutrients.

By contrast, produce that will be frozen is taken to the processing plant for flash freezing within 24 hours of harvesting. This
locks in nutrients by halting the enzymatic reactions that degrade
them.

As for canned foods, they're wonderfully convenient, and
many of them—including canned beans, corn, and pumpkin—
don't seem to suffer at all. But the heating process that's used in
canning (both to kill disease-causing microorganisms and to stop
the enzymatic degradation of nutrients) can also damage certain
phytochemicals, such as anthocyanins. If you do eat canned foods,
there are a couple things to be aware of:

- Water-soluble nutrients, such as vitamin C, leach out into the canning liquid, so use this liquid in your dish, if possible (unless you need to avoid sodium, which is often added to the liquid).
- Also, avoid fruits that are canned in heavy syrups. Those sugars will only add empty calories.

Beyond these simple precautions, says nutritionist Barbara Klein of the University of Illinois at Urbana-Champaign, it's not worth sweating the differences too much. "Eat fresh, eat frozen, eat canned," she says. "Eat whatever will get you to eat fruits and vegetables."

ELDERBERRIES

Elderberries at a Glance
- Pigments: anthocyanins (various forms of cyanidin), beta-carotene
- Other phytochemicals: quercetin, ellagic acid, catechins
- Serving size: one cup
- Vitamins and minerals per serving: C (87% of the Daily Value), A (17% DV), B_6 (17% DV), niacin (4% DV), folate (2% DV), iron (13% DV), potassium (12% DV), phosphorus (6% DV), calcium (6% DV)
- Fiber per serving: 41% DV
- ORAC score: not available

The European elderberry has been called "the medicine chest of the common people." Just about every part of the tree—leaves, flowers, berries, roots, and bark—has been used to treat one ailment or another through the years. In the 1600s, English herbalist Nicholas Culpeper wrote that the first shoots of the elder, when "boiled like asparagus, . . . do mightily carry forth phlegm and choler." And the berries, he reported, "are often given with good success to help the dropsy."

In fact, the anthocyanin-rich berries—and the wines and jams made from them—are a good source of iron and potassium. They contain 87 percent of your daily vitamin C requirement, not to mention 41 percent of the recommended fiber. No ORAC tests have been performed on fresh elderberries yet, but preliminary tests on the elderberry extracts have indicated superior antioxidant strength—and Kuresh Youdim in Jim Joseph's lab has shown that elderberry extracts help protect against oxidative stress in the type of cells that line blood vessels. (He performed these tests in the lab on cells from a cow's aorta, which serves as a good model for human cells.) This means that elderberries could play a role in protecting against heart disease and strokes. Some unpublished studies also suggest that elderberry extracts have anti-inflammatory potential.

Work in humans is scarce. But one recent study of 15 members of the 17th Austrian Armored Hunter Battalion showed that elderberry extracts could help improve performance on standard stress tests. For six days, each participant took elderberry extracts that were prepared from a special variety of elderberries with anthocyanin levels three times the average. Before starting the treatment and again at the end of the six days, the soldiers performed a stress test, involving cycling on stationary bicycles for nine minutes at different speeds. At both the start and finish of the trial, the researchers examined blood levels of various chemicals to see how the soldiers' bodies were coping with the exercise challenge. Interestingly, cells took up more glucose during exercise after the six days of elderberry treatment. That's important, because it means that cells were getting more of the fuel they needed for these spurts of activity. They also took up more ionized magnesium, which cells use to help generate energy. The study was very small, and it was not placebo controlled. But it's an intriguing beginning. Being able to burn energy efficiently is an important factor in maintaining youthful vigor.

Another study, this one in Israel, looked at the antiviral effects of elderberry extracts. During a flu outbreak on a kibbutz, 40 patients who went to the doctor within 24 hours were given either elderberry extracts or a placebo. Those who took the extracts recovered in just two or three days. Those who received the placebo took six days to recuperate. The effects need to be replicated, and larger studies need to be run. But some early lab tests from an Indiana company called Artemis International seem to confirm that elderberries can fight certain infections. "What knocks your socks off is the effect on herpes," says Artemis president Jan Mills. It will be many years before all the evidence comes together. But given the potential benefits for the heart, exercise capacity, and virus protection, how can you go wrong with anthocyanin-dense elderberries?

CONCORD GRAPES

Concord Grapes at a Glance
- Pigments: anthocyanins (various forms of cyanidin, peonidin, delphinidin, petunidin, and malvidin)
- Other phytochemicals: chlorogenic acid, caffeic acid, cinnamic acid, catechin, epicatechin, gallic acid, geraniol, p-coumaric acid, kaempferol, myricetin, quercetin, resveratrol, condensed tannins, tartaric acid
- Serving size: one cup
- Vitamins and minerals per serving: C (8% of the Daily Value), potassium (5% DV), calcium (3% DV), iron (2% DV)
- Fiber per serving: 4% DV
- ORAC score: 1,470 (for Concord grape juice; no score is available for the grapes)

So you want to be a millionaire? Just answer this question: Where were Concord grapes first bred? You won't need to call your lifelines or poll the audience to answer this one.

Concord grapes originated in Concord, Massachusetts. That's where Ephraim Wales Bull lived in the mid-1800s and where he decided to breed a strain of grapes that would grow well in chilly New England rather than the sunny climes of southern France and Italy. In 1849, after rejecting thousands of seedlings, he finally found the grape of his dreams. It had a strong, sweet flavor. More important, it was hardy, and it ripened early to escape the northern frosts. To honor his hometown, he named it the Concord grape.

Today Concord residents describe this dark blue-purple fruit in the reverent tones usually reserved for fine wines: "tart yet sweet, bold-flavored, beautifully fragrant, dusky, and deeply hued," in the words of a local writer. Despite the rhapsodic descriptions, you don't commonly find these grapes in markets. Usually they're used to make Concord grape juice and jelly. If you do see them for sale, however, buy them. They have seeds, and their thick skins are slightly bitter. But the flesh is incomparable. It's like biting into Welch's grape juice. The taste is so sweet and strong, you've never tasted another grape like it.

When it comes to antioxidant strength, too, it's hard to beat this deep purple elixir of life. The ORAC test at Tufts showed that Concord grape juice had four times the antioxidant power of other juices, including orange, tomato, and grapefruit. Perhaps that's not surprising. Look how intense the color is. Recent analyses have counted up to 31 types of anthocyanins in Concord grapes, putting them on a par with the bluest of blueberries. Those anthocyanins, together with the other polyphenols in Concord grapes, make for potent stuff. Once again, a fruit that was dismissed for years as nothing but sugar and water is suddenly looking pretty attractive, thanks to its pigments and other phytonutrients.

ANTIOXIDANT PUNCH

When Ronald Prior and Guohua Cao at Tufts tested beverages for their antioxidant strength, Concord grape juice was the hands-down winner, with antioxidant levels four times higher than any other juice. Bear in mind, however, that these scores are averages— and that wines and teas may be as potent as grape juice, depending on the grapes used (in the case of wine) or the dilution levels (for tea). By the way, sodas have almost no antioxidants at all.

Drink	ORAC
Concord grape juice	1,470*
Red wine	985
Tea	831
Grapefruit juice	359
Tomato juice	346

Drink	ORAC
Orange juice	322
Apple juice	249
White wine	196
Cranberry juice	159

*measured in ORAC points per 100 milliliters of fluid (or about 3.4 fluid ounces, just under half a cup)
Source: Ronald Prior, USDA-Agricultural Research Service

Get the Real Thing

Be sure to look for 100 percent grape juice, not grape drink. The artificial colors and flavorings in the fake stuff won't do a thing for your heart, and the corn syrup doesn't help either. Even with 100 percent grape juice, remember to watch out for calories. A 10-ounce bottle has 190.

Grape Expectations

As you might expect, all this antioxidant strength makes Concord grape juice an excellent drink for promoting heart health. That's because LDL, or "bad" cholesterol, only becomes dangerous when it's oxidized. Here's why. In the normal course of maintaining the body, cholesterol passes out of the bloodstream, through capillary walls, and into tissues that use cholesterol to build cell membranes. Similarly, it burrows into the walls of veins and arteries. If the LDL is unused, it passes back out into the bloodstream—unless it gets oxidized. Then it sticks to blood vessels, attracting the body's immune cells, which proceed to attack the interloper by swallowing it whole. When these immune cells die in the blood-vessel walls, the debris empties out into the walls. The body then recruits more immune cells to clean up the mess, and the whole process escalates, leading to inflammation and the development of plaques.

Grape juice can help break the cycle before it's too late. Together with his colleagues, John Folts, professor of medicine at the University of Wisconsin Medical School in Madison, recruited 15 adults with coronary artery disease and had them drink about

16 ounces of Concord grape juice every day for two weeks. At the beginning and again at the end of the trial, he drew a sample of blood and tested it in the lab. Not surprisingly, the grape juice reduced the susceptibility of the patients' LDL to oxidation. At the outset of the study, it took an average of 87 minutes before oxidation began. By the end, that time was up to 117 minutes—an increase of 34 percent. "If you can postpone oxidation by a significant amount, the theory is that you buy some time for LDL to get back out of the artery wall," says Folts. "People with excellent cardiovascular health usually have a slow onset of LDL oxidation."

Reducing oxidation is great. But grape juice can do far more. The flavonoids in grape juice also help keep arteries elastic. That's important, because arteries need to expand quickly in response to increased blood flow. That's the only way they can deliver enough oxygen and nutrients to the brain, muscles, and other organs when needed. In the same study, Folts found that the arteries of patients with coronary artery disease could expand only 2.2 percent in response to increased blood flow. By the end, they could expand 6.4 percent. That means that the elasticity of their blood vessels improved almost threefold in just two weeks! But this finding has even greater implications than that, because it means that the endothelial cells that line blood vessels were functioning better—and when endothelial cells are healthy, they also provide a barrier against the development of atherosclerosis.

Grape juice does one more very important thing. It turns down the activity of platelets. These are the tiny discs in the blood that are responsible for clotting. Of course, you want your blood to clot if you cut your finger. But if platelets become too active, they can cause clots to form inside blood vessels, leading to heart attacks. In a separate study, Folts asked 10 healthy volunteers to drink two cups of grape juice every day for a week. In later weeks, he asked the same volunteers to drink orange juice or grapefruit juice instead. Again, he drew blood samples at the beginning and the end of each phase and tested them in the lab for signs of platelet aggregation. Drinking purple grape juice for a week reduced platelet clumping by 77 percent. Orange and grapefruit juice had no effect.

Together, these effects could turn out to be very powerful. "These are three of the critical factors in reducing the onset of coronary artery disease," says Folts, "and grape juice seems to help all three."

Bringing Down Superoxide

Before scientists accept the results of experiments like these, however, they always need to see confirmation from other studies— and they want to know not just *that* a change is occurring, but also *why*. Cardiologist Jane Freedman at Georgetown University, in collaboration with Folts and other researchers, has helped on both accounts. In a new study, she gave 20 healthy volunteers two glasses of purple grape juice a day for two weeks. Platelet aggregation in the volunteers diminished by a third. But Freedman took the work one step further. She found that the platelets were generating almost twice as much nitric oxide as before the grape juice treatment. Since nitric oxide inhibits platelet "stickiness," that suggests that grape juice somehow boosts the ability of platelets to produce this critical molecule. That's not all. When platelets begin aggregating, they produce a nasty free radical called superoxide, which zaps beneficial nitric oxide—and probably strikes LDL, too. But Freedman found that levels of superoxide in the volunteers' blood fell by a third when they drank grape juice.

Resveratrol—Trendy and Famous

What compounds in grape juice are doing all these good things? The flavonoids have to be at least partly responsible. Folts has early evidence that the flavonoids in grape juice actually bind to LDL and travel around the body with it, providing antioxidant protection. They also seem to contribute to the elasticity of blood vessels. And Freedman has found that the condensed tannins and a subset of flavonoids called flavonols (including quercetin, kaempferol, and myricetin) are particularly effective for reducing platelet aggregation. But there are so many compounds in grape juice, it's hard to single one out. "Most fruits and vegetables have one or two groups of phenolics that they're high in," says Andrew Waterhouse, professor of enology at the University of California, Davis. By contrast, grape juice and its cousin red wine have an encyclopedia's worth. They have phenolic acids, including caffeic and gallic acids. They have tannins and condensed tannins. They have flavonoids, ranging from anthocyanins and catechins to flavonols. All of them seem to contribute to the overall antioxidant effect.

So does yet another polyphenolic compound called *resveratrol*. Grapes have more of this antioxidant than any other food that's been studied. But the levels are wildly variable. "Resveratrol is produced in response to trauma, including fungal and bacterial infections," explains James Magee, a research horticulturist at the USDA-ARS Small Fruit Research Station in Poplarville, Mississippi. As a result, levels are highest when grapes are defending themselves against these attacks. After the infection goes away, levels drop, much like human antibodies, which multiply rapidly in response to a microbial invader, then decrease when the threat has been neutralized.

Lots of media attention has focused on resveratrol, but does it live up to the hype? "It's the Julia Roberts of phenolic compounds—trendy and famous," says Waterhouse. "But it is no better an antioxidant than the hundred or so other phenolic compounds in red wine." And no evidence has shown that it is especially responsible for the heart-healthy benefits of wine and grape juice, especially since their resveratrol levels are often low. The beauty of red wine and grape juice is that you're not loading up on just one phenolic compound. There are so many, says Waterhouse, "You're hedging your bets."

Blithe Spirits

Red wine, of course, is right up there with grape juice in promoting heart health—and anyone who doubts that need only look at the evidence from France. In the early 1990s, epidemiologist Serge Renaud revealed the so-called French Paradox. The French, it seems, are able to indulge in fat-laden brie and goose-liver pâté, puff on nasty Gaulloise cigarettes, and still have less heart disease than Americans. The reason why remains open to debate. But at least one cause seems to be the *vin rouge* that the French sip with their meals. (Another is probably the large quantities of fresh fruits and vegetables they consume.)

It's hardly surprising that wine should show beneficial effects. It has the same protective phenolics as grape juice—but even more of them. "When you make grape juice, you heat the grapes to extract the flavonoids from the skins and seeds," says Folts. "But the processing only takes a day or two, and you don't get them all." By contrast, when you make red wine, the grapes ferment in vats for weeks. As the sugars turn to alcohol, the alcohol draws flavonoids and other phenolics out of the skins and seeds. To get equal amounts from grape juice and red wine, you need to drink 50 percent more juice, according to Folts. Of course, it isn't hard to drink a lot of juice. A small bottle contains 10 ounces—versus 5 ounces for a standard glass of wine.

In addition to all these phytochemicals, the alcohol in wine has a protective effect, too. It is well documented that moderate alcohol intake—from any alcoholic beverage, not just wine—produces an increase in HDL, or "good" cholesterol. "Rarely will you find such consistent evidence in the scientific literature," says Eric Rimm, associate professor of epidemiology and nutrition at Harvard. "In thirty-four studies, there was a twenty-five percent reduction of heart-disease risk on average in moderate drinkers, regardless of the source of the alcohol."

What Does "Moderate" Drinking Mean?

A drink of alcohol is defined as 12 ounces of beer, 5 ounces of wine, or 1.5 ounces of distilled spirits. Moderate alcohol consumption in turn is defined as a maximum of two drinks a day for men—or no more than one for women. "One a day" literally means one drink in a 24-hour period. You cannot save up all your daily drinks for the weekend and maintain the protective benefits.

In large doses, alcohol becomes a pro-oxidant. It kills brain cells. It causes cirrhosis of the liver. It increases a person's risks of strokes and many types of cancer—including breast, mouth, esophageal, colorectal, and liver cancers. "Next to smoking, excessive drinking is the single most risky thing we do to cause cancer," says Dr. John D. Potter of the Fred Hutchinson Cancer Research Center in Seattle. His advice: "Drink grape juice."

Red Beats White

With wines, as with every other food in this book, the most colorful ones confer the most benefits. "White wines have one-twentieth the levels of phenolics as red wines," says Leroy Creasy, professor emeritus of pomology at Cornell University. "To get the same effect from white wine, you have to drink twenty times as much." You might reasonably assume that's because red wine is made from anthocyanin-rich red grapes, while white wines come from green grapes. But you would be wrong. In fact, both come from red grapes. The difference is in the processing, but it's a crucial difference. In making white wine, the juice is pressed out of the grapes before fermentation—a process that fails to extract most of the flavonoids and other phenolics that are concentrated in the skin and seeds. In making red wine, however, the entire grape is fermented before the juice is pressed out. "Everything in the skin is extracted out by the alcohol," says Creasy. Rosé wines are somewhere in the middle. The skins and seeds are left in the vat part of the time, with mid-range results in extraction of phenols and flavonoids.

Cancer-Proofing Galore

So far, nobody has found wine or grape juice to be a cancer fighter. But a phytochemical that's found in both could be. That's resveratrol. John Pezzuto, associate dean of the college of pharmacy at the University of Illinois at Chicago, has found that it can intervene in various ways to prevent tumor growth. At the outset, it stimulates detoxification enzymes. In this way, resveratrol helps neutralize carcinogens before they can lead to mutations.

But one or two mutations alone are not enough to cause cancer, particularly if they're in strands of "junk" DNA that serve no known purpose. For an abnormal cell to become cancerous, other things must happen to it, too. For instance, cancer-causing oncogenes must be turned on and tumor suppressor genes turned off. Resveratrol steps in again to prevent abnormal cells from transforming themselves into cancerous ones by sopping up free radicals and preventing inflammation. (Like curcumin, resveratrol is a potent COX-2 inhibitor, an important type of anti-inflammatory.) Pezzuto found that he could halve the number of breast cancers in rats by feeding the animals resveratrol—and totally prevent skin tumors in mice.

Finally, resveratrol tackles any full-fledged cancer cells that may emerge and helps wrestle them into normalcy by encouraging something called cell differentiation. To understand why differentiation matters, let's step back briefly to the moment of conception. In a human embryo, all cells are identical. These cells divide and multiply rapidly in a headlong dash toward personhood. But along the way, they must develop identities as skin cells, liver cells, heart cells, brain cells, and so on. Otherwise, a person would never develop out of this mush. Once a cell is fully "differentiated," there are tight limits on how it can behave and how rapidly it can multiply. But for reasons that are not fully understood, cancer cells do not fully differentiate. That means they are able to multiply rapidly, as if they were embryos, and solid tumors may form as the cells pile up on top of one another. Pezzuto was able to take leukemia cells in the lab and, using resveratrol, make them differentiate into cells that behaved normally. "Resveratrol shows real promise," he concludes. "It's being evaluated now by the National Cancer Institute in preclinical testing."

Of course, there's not enough resveratrol in the diet to serve in lieu of chemotherapy—and drinking large amounts of cancer-promoting alcohol would defeat the purpose. "But it's conceivable that in combination with other phytochemicals in the diet, it could help with cancer prevention," says Pezzuto.

RAISINS

Raisins at a Glance
- Pigments: oxidized sugars, oxidized cinnamic acids
- Phytochemicals: quercetin, rutin, kaempferol, caftaric acid, coutaric acid, tartaric acid, inulin
- Serving size: one-quarter cup
- Vitamins and minerals per serving: iron (6% of the Daily Value), calcium (2% DV), potassium (8% DV), thiamin (4% DV), riboflavin (2% DV), B_6 (5% DV)
- Fiber per serving: 9% DV
- ORAC score: 2,830

The first raisins were probably grapes that dried naturally on the vine—or perhaps grapes that fell on the ground and shriveled in the sun. Either way, they tasted good enough that people quickly learned to make these sweet morsels deliberately. As long as 3,000 years ago, historians tell us, ancient Egyptians were laying out grapes in the sun to dry. Raisins were so highly valued that they became a form of currency in countries bordering the Mediterranean. In ancient Israel, citizens used them to pay taxes. In ancient Rome, where breakfast often consisted of bread with a few raisins, two jars of the precious commodity could purchase a slave.

Today, raisins aren't used as money, but they're worth their weight in antioxidants. Since raisins are dried grapes, it's hardly surprising that they pack a wallop of an antioxidant punch. Grapes themselves have high ORAC scores, but once you eliminate the water from the fruit, you're left with a more concentrated dose of antioxidants and other polyphenolics. That's also why, ounce for ounce, raisins have higher vitamin and mineral concentrations than grapes—and more calories, too.

But there is at least one thing you'll find in raisins that does not appear to be in grapes. It's a fiberlike carbohydrate called *inulin*. "It basically consists of lots of fructose molecules linked together," says Mary Ellen Camire, professor of food science and human nutrition at the University of Maine. "We think there's something about the drying process that makes those sugars come together as inulin." Like the fructooligosaccharides in bananas, inulin is a favored food of the beneficial bacteria in the gut. These bacteria help prevent food-borne infections such as *E. coli* and salmonella, and they keep populations of diarrhea-causing bacteria under control. When inulin ferments, it also produces short-chain fatty acids that help lower cholesterol. "When the colon senses the buildup of fatty acids, it sends a message to the liver to stop making cholesterol," says Camire.

There are still more ways that raisins contribute to colon health. Gene Spiller, founder of the Health Research and Studies Center in Los Altos, California, has shown that the fiber and tartaric acid in raisins combine to speed food and waste through and to decrease the bile acids that may contribute to colon cancer. Just one small box a day is enough to help, he says—provided the rest of your diet is good.

By the way, just as red and white wines both start as red

grapes, dark and golden raisins both come from green grapes—
generally Thompson Seedless grapes, which are also the most popular green grapes for eating in this country. The difference
between the two raisins is in the processing. Dark raisins are dried
on paper trays that are laid out in the sun. During that sun drying,
sugars and amino acids link and turn brown. At the same time,
enzymes cause many of the polyphenolic compounds to oxidize,
producing browning as well (just as oxidation turns tea from
green to black). By contrast, golden raisins are dehydrated in a
drying tunnel with a fan that blows hot, dry air over them for 16
to 18 hours. They are treated first with a blast of sulfur dioxide
gas to prevent browning reactions.

As with tea, the difference between oxidized and unoxidized
polyphenolics means that the content of dark and golden raisins is
somewhat different. Which is better? "It's too early to say," says
Ronald Wrolstad of Oregon State University, who has analyzed
the polyphenolics in raisins. "All we can say at this point is they're
different." But a word to the wise. Because golden raisins are
treated with sulfur dioxide, anyone who's allergic to sulfites
should avoid them.

EGGPLANT

Eggplant at a Glance
- Pigments: anthocyanins (various forms of delphinidin)
- Other phytochemicals: caffeic acid, chlorogenic acid, tan-
  nins, saponins
- Serving size: one-half cup
- Vitamins and minerals per serving: Folate (2% of the Daily
  Value), B_6 (2% DV), potassium (3% DV), copper (3% DV),
  iron (1% DV)
- Fiber per serving: 5% DV
- ORAC: 390

Eggplants have been cultivated in China and India since the
fifth century. In the 12th century, Arabs introduced them into
Spain. Although the Spaniards loved them, other Europeans were

slow to accept them, for fear that they caused madness, bad breath, leprosy, and cancer. With a reputation like that, no wonder the plant was relegated to an ornamental role! Today, we might not think of eggplants as decorative, but the first ones that English speakers encountered seem to have been white, egg-shaped fruits. The image of eggs growing on miniature trees must have held a certain charm.

Eggplants are not the richest source of vitamins or phytochemicals. Maybe that's because the deeply pigmented purple is only on the outside—and we generally don't eat the skins. Eggplant does, however, contain a class of phytochemicals known as saponins. No one has specifically studied the saponins in eggplant, but studies have suggested that the saponins in legumes have antihistaminic, antioxidant, and anti-inflammatory properties. In addition, they can help lower cholesterol rates by binding with cholesterol and bile acids in the gut and ushering these out of the body.

Eggplants also contain a nice amount of cholesterol-lowering pectin. And James Duke, author of *The Green Pharmacy*, reports that eggplant contains four substances that help fight asthma by reducing bronchial spasms. So do tomatoes. Bell peppers and onions have five apiece. Put those together and you'll have a pretty healthy ratatouille. You'll find a recipe on page 267.

Banish Wrinkles

We've spent a lot of this book discussing cancer and heart disease. But what about a problem that people *really* spend time fretting about?—skin wrinkling. There is new evidence that eggplant, when eaten as part of a diet rich in fruits and vegetables, may help prevent this scourge of aging. An international team of researchers performed a preliminary study among 453 people in Sweden, Greece, and Australia. In each population, certain foods—such as whole milk, red meat, butter, sodas, and pastries—were associated with greater skin damage. By contrast, people with less wrinkled skin ate diets that could have come straight out of *The Color Code*. These regimens were heavy on vegetables (spinach, leafy greens, eggplant, asparagus, celery, onions, leeks, and garlic), fruits (cherries, grapes, melon, prunes, and apples), and finally eggs, yogurt, nuts, olives, tea, and legumes. This makes a lot of sense, because fruits and vegetables are loaded with antioxidants—and most skin damage is the result of oxidative stress caused when sunlight strikes the skin.

As the authors of the study wrote: "There is growing evidence that the important antioxidants in human diets are much more than the vitamins C, E, or beta-carotene. . . . Due to their antioxidant activity, polyphenols present in plant food such as tea, apples, onions, garlic, and eggplant appear to be partially responsible for many of the protective effects against oxidative stress of the skin."

GETTING THE MOST OUT OF YOUR EGGPLANT

Eggplant has a meaty texture that works well for a variety of vegetarian entreés. The problem is that eggplant tends to soak up a lot of oil in cooking. That's why Elizabeth Ward of the American Dietetic Association avoids oil altogether when she prepares eggplant. Instead she peels and slices it, then dips the slices first in skim milk and then in bread crumbs. Finally she bakes the eggplant in the oven. "Otherwise, for all the fat you've put on it, it's sort of like taking potatoes and making them into French fries," she says. If you do use oil, make it a healthy olive oil.

NOTE: Many chefs salt eggplant before cooking to draw out water and eliminate the slightly bitter taste. Unfortunately, this will also neutralize the beneficial saponins, which cause that bitterness.

PLUMS AND DRIED PLUMS (PRUNES)

Plums at a Glance
- Pigments: anthocyanins (various forms of cyanidin), beta-carotene
- Other phytochemicals: chlorogenic acid, p-coumaric acid, ferulic acid, malic acid
- Serving size: 2 medium plums
- Vitamins and minerals per serving: A (9% of the Daily Value), C (20% DV), riboflavin (7% DV), thiamin (6% DV), potassium (7% DV), magnesium (3% DV)

- Fiber per serving: 8% DV
- ORAC: 949

Plums have long been prized. So exceptional is their image that their name has become synonymous with desirability. Today, a "plum" job is a very attractive one. When it comes to nutrition, plums are pretty attractive, too. They are a good source of vitamin C and offer an excellent supply of other vitamins and minerals. And they really shine when it comes to ORAC testing. With a score of 949, they're among the top ten fresh fruits. Of course, a lot of that antioxidant power comes from the purple pigments in their skins.

The main reason why plums are not more popular today is that they are often somewhat bitter. In the late 1800s, botanist Luther Burbank attempted to solve this problem by crossing a plum and an apricot. The sugar content of the apricots gave his hybrids greater sweetness—and the apricots' beta-carotene boosted carotenoids, too. Lately, new plum-apricot hybrids have started appearing on shop shelves with intriguing, trademarked names like Dinosaur Eggs, Pluots, and Plumcots. Like other plums, they are ready for eating when they yield to slight pressure but have no obvious soft spots.

Dried Plums (Prunes) at a Glance

- Pigments: anthocyanins (various forms of cyanidin)
- Other phytochemicals: chlorogenic acid, *p*-coumaric acid, ferulic acid, malic acid, sorbitol
- Serving size: 5 dried plums
- Vitamins and minerals per serving: A (17% of the Daily Value), C (3% DV), niacin (4% DV), potassium (9% DV), iron (6% DV), calcium (2% DV)
- Fiber per serving: 12% DV
- ORAC: 5,770

Even prune lovers admit it: Prunes have an image problem. That's why the California Prune Board recently changed its name to the California Dried Plum Board. But despite the image polishing, the unglamorous fact remains. Prunes, as our grandmothers used to say, are "good for what ails you." With generous amounts of fiber plus a natural sugar called sorbitol that soaks up water, they are an excellent bulking agent to get the intestinal *plumb*ing working again. Maybe they should call them "dried plumbs."

No name tinkering, however, can gild the fruit's image as much as the ORAC tests at Tufts have. Of all the fruits and vegetables tested, prunes came out on top, with a record-smashing 5,770 points. Not bad for a wrinkled old fruit that Grannie touted, eh? If antioxidants really can help slow aging, as some experts claim, then prunes (excuse us, dried plums) are perfectly positioned to become a star in the firmament of anti-aging foods. Of course, part of the reason they shot to the top of the ORAC chart is that they're dried, giving them an unfair advantage in any ounce-for-ounce comparison. Without water to weigh them down, the antioxidants are more concentrated—and so are the calorie-laden sugars. Still, the purple plums they come from have a top-ten ORAC score of 949, which isn't too shabby either. Once again, blue-purple foods rule!

LAVENDER

In trendy New York restaurants, a new herb has crept onto menus lately—lavender. From lavender-garnished salads to lavender-melon soup, the herb is adding a whiff of perfumed elegance to many a repast. You may have encountered the flavor before in lavender-scented Violet candies or in the herbal mixture called Herbes de Provence—or maybe you haven't run across it at all. But everyone who tries it seems to agree that a soupçon of lavender adds a certain *je ne sais quoi* to a meal.

The reason for including lavender isn't just the novelty of using a purple herb. The essential oil that gives lavender its flowery essence is chock full of beneficial phytochemicals. One of the most important is perillyl alcohol, which has attracted attention lately as a promising cancer fighter. Because perillyl alcohol both slows the division of cancer cells and also encourages them to self-destruct, it fights tumor growth in two important ways. "There isn't much perillyl alcohol in the diet," says Michael Gould, professor of oncology at the University of Wisconsin Medical School in Madison. Lavender is one of the few sources. "French perfume chemists discovered perillyl alcohol at the turn of the last century, while trying to find out what made a hybrid lavender smell nice," he says. Of course, a sprig of lavender on your plate won't deliver phamarcologic doses of perillyl alcohol, but the trace that you do obtain is yet another component of an all-round cancer-fighting diet.

Cooking with Lavender

If you try cooking with lavender, do not use dried lavender from potpourri or sachets, which often contain added perfumes. Lavender at the florist's also may be treated with chemicals that render it inedible. Instead, buy lavender at a greengrocer's or grow it yourself. Some chefs claim that the best varieties for cooking are the English Hidcote and Munstead or the French hybrid lavendin. Hidcote has particularly dark purple flowers and an intense flavor. Deep purple is good!

THE COLOR CODE
EATING PROGRAM

"The preservation of health is a *duty*. Few seem conscious
that there is such a thing as physical morality."
—Herbert Spencer (1820–1903)

AMERICANS SEEM CONSTANTLY TO BE ON DIETS—grapefruit
diets, cabbage diets, low-carb diets, high-protein diets, raw food
diets, you name it. The elusive goal of these many plans is weight
loss. Yet we have the fattest society ever.

Forget these crazy schemes.

The original Greek word for diet was *diaita*, meaning a "way
of life." That is a perfect description of the Color Code eating
plan. It's a way of life that revels in the glorious spectrum of color
that nature has provided us in foods. It's also a way of life that
confers innumerable health benefits.

Now that you know what many of these benefits are, we will
share with you our easy plan to build colorful fruits and vegetables into your diet. You'll be glad to know that you don't have to
give up anything you love. There are no forbidden foods in the
Color Code eating program. As we see it, the inevitable result of
depriving people of tasty meals is merely to send them to the
supermarket two weeks later in search of junk food. That's why
there are no *don'ts* in this eating program. Only *do's*. But if you
follow the guidelines, the good foods will gradually start to edge
out the less healthful choices. Fruit snacks will replace donuts. Tea
will oust sodas. Pretty soon, you'll be living a healthier life. Mary
Fleming, a dietician in Maine who works with Dan Nadeau, has
seen extremely positive results when she put patients on the pro-

gram. "It's an exciting and easy plan that makes healthy eating fun," she says.

GO FOR THE GOLD

The starting point of this eating plan is a simple color scoring system. There are no cumbersome calorie counts here—just an easy plan to make sure you're getting enough fruits and vegetables from the different color categories. Your goal here is to strive for a daily "color score" of 100 points. The most important way to earn these points is simply to eat fruits and vegetables, but there are easy ways to earn bonus points, too. We'll provide dozens of tips to help you. Ready?

Your Plan for Color Scoring

There is only one essential rule to remember: **Eat 9 to 10 servings of fruits and vegetables a day. Points: 10 each.**

"Wait a minute!" you say. "What about the Five a Day program? Aren't people supposed to eat five servings of fruits and vegetables a day?" Well, yes. But the USDA Food Guide Pyramid actually prescribes a total of five to *nine* servings a day—that is, three to five servings of vegetables and an additional two to four of fruit. The greatest benefits are at the top end of that range. "Of course, we know that people should eat nine servings a day," admits Barbara Berry of the Produce for Better Health Foundation, which runs the Five a Day campaign, together with the National Cancer Institute. "But people aren't even eating five. You have to start somewhere."

Programs with serious health improvement goals have even more radical targets. The DASH diet, which aims to reduce high blood pressure, prescribes 10 servings of fruits and vegetables a day. The experimental cancer-prevention diet at the AMC Cancer Research Center in Denver calls for 10 to 16.

The Good News

Right now, you may be saying to yourself, "No way! I can't eat nine to ten servings a day of that stuff every day." But here's the good news. You're probably eating more than you realize already. It isn't really that hard if you keep these tips in mind:

- *Remember that serving sizes aren't that big.* Half a cup of chopped raw vegetables or fruit makes a serving. Half a cup may sound like a lot, but it isn't. That's about the amount that would fill half a baseball. And a baseball fills up quickly, when you're talking about water-laden fruit. For dried fruit, a serving size is even smaller—a quarter cup, or the size of a small box of raisins. Here is a general guide to serving sizes for fruits:

  > Large fruit (cantaloupe, pineapple): 1 slice
  > Medium fruit (apple, orange, banana): 1 fruit
  > Small fruit (plums, kiwis, clementines): 2 fruits
  > Berries (blueberries, strawberries): 1 cup
  > Dried fruit (dried apricots, figs): ¼ cup

  Similarly, vegetable sizes are not large. Half a cup of chopped vegetables makes a serving. The exception is leafy greens. Because they take up so much space, a serving size is a whole cup, chopped.
- *Think in threes.* Nine servings sounds much more manageable if you think of it as three groups of three—three servings in the morning, three in the afternoon, and three at night. For example, to get to three servings in the morning, start with a glass of orange juice, and you've already knocked one off. Toss a handful of raisins into your cereal, and that's serving number two. A slice of melon on the side puts you up to three. That's three servings before you even walk out the door. Even Monopoly was never this easy! And once you start learning colorful new recipes for vegetable fajitas and stews, soups and salads, and fruit smoothies, you will quickly realize how many dishes count as two to three servings all by themselves.
- *Remember that snacks count, too.* When we were growing up, the experts discouraged snacking. Now you can relegate that old idea to the compost heap of history. The body and brain rely on glucose for fuel. By eating smaller meals and snacking a couple times a day, you can keep your body

and brain amply and steadily supplied. If, on the other hand, you go for long periods without eating, you're encouraging your body to raid its stores of protein to make glucose. (Besides, as dieters know all too well, if you skip meals, your body tries to conserve calories by slowing down your metabolism!) So go ahead and munch on an apple, some carrot sticks, or a handful of dried apricots.

- *Juices count also.* Wash down lunch with a V8 or throw some carrots into the juicer, and you get credit for a serving of produce. Fully 90 percent of the antioxidants in fruits are in the juice. Be aware, though, that when you drink juice, you sacrifice the healthy fiber in the whole fruit, along with many of the beneficial phytonutrients in the skins. And you can quickly take in too many calories, simply because you can easily guzzle, say, two glasses of apple juice instead of munching a single apple. So choose your juices carefully—avoid sugar-laced "fruit drinks"—and don't rely on them to fill your quota.

Portion Distortion

In this land of plenty, it seems that the standard serving size is now extra large. "Foreigners coming to this country express amazement at the amount of food served up in American homes and eateries," says Melanie Polk, director of nutrition education at the American Institute for Cancer Research. The "small" popcorn buckets in movie theaters used to be called "regular" a generation ago. A small ice cream cone today is often two scoops—a size that we used to call "double." Even the standard restaurant plate size has grown, says Polk—from 10.5 inches in diameter to 12 inches today. Not surprisingly, our mental image of normal serving sizes has grown, too.

But while restaurant portions have mushroomed, the USDA's definition of a serving has not. The amount of food that the USDA considers a serving is much smaller than most Americans imagine. Some examples:

- A serving of meat is three ounces, or the size of a deck of cards.
- A serving of hard cheese is one ounce, or about the size of your thumb.

- A serving of grains is one ounce. But bagels, for example, often weigh three to five ounces. That means you can get three to five servings of grains in a single helping!
- A serving of spaghetti is a half cup of cooked pasta—or 32 meager strands.
- A serving of French fries consists of just 10 fries!

"Patients tell me they couldn't possibly eat six to eleven servings of grains a day, as the USDA recommends," says dietician Elizabeth Ward of the American Dietetic Association. "I tell them, 'Oh, I bet you eat that much by two P.M.' " Ward coined the term "portion distortion" to characterize this problem of perceptions.

The good news is that portions of fruits and vegetables are also much smaller than you expect. Just six spears of asparagus make a half-cup serving of vegetables. Eight medium strawberries count as a serving of fruit. Given the hefty amounts of vitamin C, folate, and dietary fiber in those few berries—and a mere 45 calories—that's not a bad deal!

Drink to Your Health

Man, as they say, does not live by bread alone. Drinks are essential, too. But which ones? John Weisburger of the American Health Foundation has devised a "fluids pyramid" resembling the USDA's food pyramid. At the broad base is water, the most essential of fluids, which helps just about every health-preserving process in the body. "Water is more essential than food," says Weisburger. "Every enzyme in the body works in a solution of water." He recommends at least four 8-ounce glasses a day.

In the middle tier of the pyramid, at five to eight 4-ounce servings a day, Weisburger places low-calorie or no-calorie liquids such as vegetable broth and tea. Drink brewed teas if you want the full benefits. "Even children can benefit from the antioxidants in tea," says Weisburger, "but they should stick with decaffeinated tea."

On the next shelf up the pyramid—at one to two glasses a day—Weisburger places fruit and vegetable juices, such as orange juice and V8. They deliver all the great health benefits we've discussed in this book, but because they also have plenty of calories, you need to limit the proportion of your fluids that comes from juice. Soy milk and skim milk are also on this shelf of the pyramid. Note that some brands of soy milk are now fortified with calcium and vitamin D, for those who cannot digest cow's milk.

At the very top of the pyramid—the part labeled "Use Sparingly"—is red wine. Sure, it benefits the heart, but experts recommend no more than one glass a day for women and a maximum of two for men, or else any potential benefits will quickly dissipate.

SCORING BONUS POINTS

THE COLOR CODE TOP TEN LISTS

We've never met a fruit or vegetable we didn't like, but some deliver more nutritional punch than others. Here are our top ten picks for fruits and vegetables that promote health. They include high-antioxidant foods, proven disease fighters, and foods from every color group.

Fruits	Vegetables
Red:	
1. Strawberries	1. Tomatoes
2. Raspberries	2. Red bell peppers
Orange-Yellow:	
3. Oranges	3. Carrots
4. Mangoes	4. Sweet potatoes
5. Grapefruit	5. Winter squash
Green:	
6. Kiwi	6. Kale
7. Avocado	7. Broccoli
	8. Spinach
Blue-Purple:	
8. Blueberries	9. Purple cabbage
9. Concord grapes	10. Eggplant
10. Dried plums	

If you're an exceptionally good eater, you can get to your daily "color" goal of 100 points by eating ten servings of fruits and vegetables. But if you can't manage that many, don't despair. There are bonus strategies to help nudge you toward the top. If you're already at the top, you can use the bonus points to reward yourself with "extra credit." Here are our additional strategies:

- **Choose fruits and vegetables from the Color Code Top Ten lists. Bonus points: 5 each.** Wait, don't panic! We're not asking you to eat more fruits and vegetables than you've eaten already. You've already collected 10 points for each serving. Now go back and see if any of them are on these Top Ten lists. For each one that is, collect an additional 5 points.

- **Cover all four color groups in a day. Bonus points: 5.** Again, this doesn't refer to eating more; it just rewards you for consuming a *variety* of foods. Variety is really the key to a healthy eating program. Blueberries are great. But if you eat only blueberries, you'll miss out on the ellagic acid in strawberries. Focus on strawberries, and you'll miss the limonene in oranges. Bank on oranges, and you've neglected the quercetin in apples or the resveratrol in grapes. You don't need to get hung up on all the phytochemical names—just go for the whole color spectrum every day.

- **Drink tea. Bonus points: 5 for two cups.** Brewed tea delivers more ORAC points than most fruits and vegetables. Research indicates that its potent antioxidants make this beverage a super heart protector.

- **Eat a fruit or vegetable you haven't eaten in the last year. Bonus points: 5.** Often our tastes are formulated as children. Even as adults, we don't necessarily give "yucky" vegetables a second chance. That's too bad. What if Grandma overcooked the Brussels sprouts when you were a kid, or your mother never seasoned those frozen veggies? You might be missing out on vegetables you would actually love today. Brussels sprouts can be delicious if cooked to crisp-tender or soaked first in a subtle marinade. Try them again. Or sample a completely new food, like passion fruit, that wasn't widely available when you were younger. Any way you slice it, the broader your fruit-and-vegetable "repertoire," the more phytochemical protection you get.

Now Here's the Real Bonus

In addition to fighting aging, readers who follow the Color Code eating plan can lose weight and trim fat. The plan isn't a weight-loss program per se, but that's an inevitable outcome of replacing French fries and junk food with fresh fruits and vegetables. Gram for gram, produce has fewer calories and much less fat. Blueberries contain just 80 calories per cup. If you wanted to reach 2,000 calories by eating blueberries, you'd have to consume 25 cups! That means that if you eat mainly fruits, vegetables, and whole grains, you can eat a lot of food—and actually lose weight! That won't happen, of course, if you only add a glass of juice and handful of raisins to a diet of Big Macs. But if you go all the way and actually shift to a semi-vegetarian diet, the challenge won't be cutting calories. It will be getting *enough* calories.

Challenge Yourself to Eat More Colorful Foods

When it comes to food, let color be your guide, as you aim to make your meals more multi-hued than a Benetton ad. (No cheating by using artificially colored jelly beans or snack foods!)

Here are some suggestions to get you started:

- Look for recipes that combine at least two colorful foods, preferably from two different color groups. There are plenty of delicious recipes in the back of the book to choose from. But why stop there? Look up unusual fruits and vegetables like starfruit or broccoli rabe on the Internet for more great recipe ideas.
- Attend vegetarian cooking classes.
- When you're in the produce section of the supermarket, challenge yourself to find something appetizing from every color group. The Color Code Top Ten lists give you a good place to start.
- Buy a fruit or vegetable you've never eaten before. Then check the Internet for recipes or serving ideas.

- When you're cooking, see how many colors you can add to dishes. For example, there's no need for a salad to be plain green. Add carrots, red onions, purple cabbage, or any other colorful vegetable that appeals to you. And don't limit yourself to vegetables. Some salads are delicious with fruits, including mandarin oranges, strawberries, and even blueberries. Dried fruits, such as cranberries and raisins, also can be fabulous.
- Cook with colorful spices, such as turmeric and paprika.
- Use colorful garnishes, including parsley, chives, and cilantro. Color definitely adds to the visual appeal of a dish—which in turn makes it even more appetizing. Watch cooking shows for ideas, and pay attention to the color on your plate when you dine out—some chefs are very creative.
- Host a potluck dinner at your house and ask the guests to bring their most colorful recipes.
- Eat at ethnic restaurants to see how they prepare fruits and vegetables. One excellent option is a Mongolian barbecue, if there is one in your area. You start by filling your bowl at a salad bar with a wide range of colorful vegetables, plus noodles, chicken, and seafood. You then choose a mild or spicy sauce and the chef tosses everything onto a flat grill for flash cooking. At the end, you can add extra toppings, such as peanuts or fresh dill. Come back time and again to try different combinations of colorful vegetables and sauces.
- Make your snacks more colorful, too. Snacks are a terrific opportunity to abolish junk food and substitute healthful, colored foods, such as dried fruits or blueberry smoothies.

You Say "Tomato," Your Kids Say "Not!" Getting to Yes.

Getting your children to eat right can be more frustrating than getting them to clean their rooms. One friend tells us that the only thing standing between her son and malnutrition is Sesame Street vitamins. If this sounds familiar, try these tips. It's never too early to start eating right. Most chronic diseases take decades to build up—and the beginnings of atherosclerosis have been detected in children as young as eight and nine!

- Take the kids to a farmers' market and ask them to help select produce. It's hard to resist a barrel full of fresh peaches, corn, or vine-ripened tomatoes. The kids may even be tempted to eat some!

- Better yet, take them to a farm or orchard where they can pick their own fresh apples, strawberries, or blueberries.
- Be sneaky. The book *Stealth Health* by Evelyn Tribole is full of ways to disguise healthy ingredients in delicious dishes, right down to blending tofu into cheesecake.
- If the kids like frozen drinks, they'll love fruit smoothies. Make them with a variety of fresh fruits—strawberries, bananas, peaches, and, of course, blueberries—or buy frozen organic fruit without syrup. Let your kids help you make the smoothie; even very young children enjoy standing on a stool and dropping strawberries into the blender.
- Chop up fruit and leave it in the refrigerator for snacks in single-serving, reusable containers. Older kids or teens won't cut up cantaloupe on their own, but if it's already in chunks, they might grab it from the fridge.
- If oranges seem too hard for kids to peel, stock up on clementines and tangerines when they're in season. The skins peel off easily, and the fruits don't have a lot of bothersome seeds to irritate the kids.
- Serve dips. You'd be surprised how many vegetables will go down with a low-fat sauce, such as a yogurt-based dip.
- Add a spoonful of Parmesan cheese. "Kids are natural vegetable haters," says Elizabeth Ward of the American Dietetic Association. "But a little cheese on steamed cauliflower seems to take the edge off." Cheese is an intense source of calcium, and kids love it.
- Be creative. Vegetable plates can be laid out to look like people, teddy bears, or kittens. Use almonds for eyes, carrot curls for hair, and jicama slices for eyeglass arms. Make a bag of "coins" out of carrots and radishes. Fill a celery stick with peanut butter and top it with raisins to make "ants on a log." Create radish "roses" by making a series of vertical cuts around the outside.
- Play with your fruit, too. Nutritionist Melanie Polk of the American Institute for Cancer Research used to make "banana faces" for her daughter. "Start with banana slices to make the eyes, nose, teeth, mouth, and hair," says Polk.

Use raisins for the pupils or to fashion a raisin mustache. Peach slices can be ears. "To this day my daughter, who's in college, still asks for banana faces," she says.

- Plan "ethnic" food nights. Not only do kids learn about new foods and cuisines, but they can also have a lot of fun. Eat Chinese food with chopsticks. Dip pita bread into Turkish appetizers. Scoop up Ethiopian food in a flatbread called *injera*. In India, the traditional way of eating is . . . with your fingers! To do it properly, have fingerbowls handy and do not get your fingers dirty above the second knuckle.
- And finally, set a good example. If you eat fruits and vegetables, your kids are more likely to do the same.

ROUNDING OUT YOUR PLATE

Obviously, it takes more than fruits and vegetables to make a well-rounded diet. The discovery of phytochemicals may herald the dawn of a new age in nutrition. But as wonderful as fruits and vegetables are, they occupy only the middle third of the USDA Food Guide Pyramid. The broad base of the pyramid—the foundation of a healthy diet—is filled with grains, including bread, cereal, rice, and pastas. Dan Nadeau tells his patients to think in terms of dinner plates. Overall, whole grains should make up half the plate. Another 30 to 40 percent should be vegetables and fruits (including dessert). The other 10 to 20 percent should be split between proteins—that is, legumes, fish, and fowl.

Here are our recommendations for rounding out the rest of your plate in as healthful a way as possible.

Reap the Benefits of Whole Grains
Believe it or not, you can reduce your risks of diabetes, stroke, heart disease, and various cancers by simply substituting whole grains for refined ones. That means shopping for brown rice rather than white or for dense, tasty, whole-wheat bread rather than the squishy, bland, white stuff. What's the advantage? The fiber in wheat is mainly concentrated in the bran, or outer coating of the kernel. A vast storehouse of vitamins and minerals is in the

germ, or embryo—including selenium, magnesium, thiamin, phosphorus, zinc, and vitamin E. But these are precisely the parts that are stripped away in making refined white flours and white rice. You're being cheated out of all these nutrients!

The Nurses' Health Study recently found that those who ate the most whole grains—close to three servings a day—reduced their stroke risk by 43 percent. The Iowa Women's Health Study found that women who ate the most whole grains and cereal fiber reduced their risks of diabetes by 20 percent. It also found that at least one serving of whole grains a day reduced the women's risk of dying at all during a nine-year period by 15 percent. "Most of that effect came from reducing heart disease, since that's the leading cause of death," says Lawrence Kushi, a nutritional epidemiologist at Columbia University. "But reduced cancer rates also played a role."

HOW CAN YOU FIND WHOLE GRAINS?

Finding whole grains isn't always as easy as it sounds. Just because a bread is brown, that doesn't make it whole wheat; breads can be colored with caramel or molasses. The name on the label can be equally misleading. Words like "stone ground," "organic," and even "seven grain" do not necessarily guarantee a whole-grain product.

There are two ways to tell for sure:

- First, turn to the list of ingredients. The very first ingredient should include the word "whole." It if doesn't, then it's not a whole-grain product. Settle for nothing less than the "whole" package. This goes for any and all baked goods—bread, crackers, breakfast cereals, pretzels, you name it.
- Second, look on the "Nutrition Facts" label for a fiber content of two to four grams per serving. If it's got less, it's too refined.

In addition to searching out whole-grain breads and cereals, you can buy minimally processed grains, such as brown rice, barley, and oats.

Use the Old Bean

Legumes could help you avoid heart disease and maybe even cancer. These foods—including peas, green beans, lentils, chickpeas, and black beans—aren't technically considered vegetables. Their main claim to dietary fame is that they are significant sources of protein. In past years, however, the thinking was that they provided "incomplete" protein, meaning that they did not supply all nine essential amino acids. That thinking is now considered passé. "The terms 'complete' and 'incomplete' are a misnomer," says Mark Messina, associate professor of nutrition at Loma Linda University. "Some legumes are higher or lower in certain amino acids, but they have them all." It's still a good idea to eat foods like rice and beans that balance out the protein mix, but there's no need to eat them together.

There's one more advantage to eating legumes. In addition to protein, you'll get hefty doses of fiber and folate. Lentils are particularly high in both. Folate helps rid your body of heart-disease–causing homocysteine. A new study from the Mayo Clinic suggests that it also reduces breast cancer risk in women who put themselves at increased risk by drinking more than four grams of alcohol a day (half a drink). Researchers are not sure why folate helps, but they think it may improve the body's ability to repair DNA breaks caused by alcohol. Fiber, too, helps prevent a number of diseases, including diabetes. Put them together and you've got a major disease-fighting food. In the Adventist Health Study, legumes stood out as a protective factor against colon cancer.

Haul in a Fish Dish

For starters, fish is a terrific source of protein. But that is not the only reason to eat it. Fish—particularly oily fish like salmon, mackerel, sardines, and tuna—are low in saturated fat, but rich in omega-3 fatty acids. Despite the dreaded word "fatty," these polyunsaturated fats are beneficial, even essential, since the human body cannot make them for itself. The omega-3s help quiet inflammation and prevent overaggressive platelet clumping in the blood. The Nurses' Health Study recently found that women who ate fish once a week cut their risk of stroke by 22 percent, while

BE A BEAN COUNTER

There are many ways to get protein in your diet. But if you get your protein from legumes, you'll also get folate and fiber. Soybeans are an exceptional source of high-quality protein—"better than red meat," says Leonard Cohen of the American Health Foundation. Lentils are high in all three—protein, fiber, and folate. A 2,000-calorie diet should include at least 25 grams of fiber and 400 micrograms of folate.

Legume	Protein*	Dietary Fiber*	Folate**
Soybeans	14	5	46
Lentils	9	8	179
White beans	9	6	72
Split peas	8	8	64
Black beans	8	7	128
Kidney beans	8	6	114
Pinto beans	7	7	147
Chickpeas	7	6	141
Lima beans	7	7	78

*measured in grams per half cup of cooked beans
**measured in micrograms per half cup of cooked beans

those who dined on fish five or more times a week slashed the odds of stroke by 52 percent. Because the evidence is now so clear that omega-3s promote heart health, the American Heart Association recently changed its guidelines to recommend that all adults eat fish twice a week. (The FDA, however, recently warned pregnant women against four types of fish with high mercury levels—shark, swordfish, tilefish, and king mackerel.)

In addition to soothing hearts, these oils appear to be crucial to normal brain functioning. A series of crossnational studies has linked low fish consumption to a range of psychiatric disorders, from major depression and bipolar disorder to postpartum depression and suicidal tendencies. Only 40 percent of Americans get enough omega-3 oils in their diets. (The long-chain omega-3s are found almost exclusively in seafood. But shorter-chain omega-3 fatty acids are also found in walnuts, flaxseed, canola oil, and dark greens, such as spinach and kale.)

Slip in Some Healthy Oils, Such as Olive and Canola

Balsamic vinaigrette made with extra-virgin olive oil can be exquisite on a salad. Nothing else rivals the taste—and it's so good for you. Olive oil is richer than any other oil in monounsaturated fatty acids, which help raise "good" cholesterol. More than 70 percent of its fats are this heart-healthy type. Olive oil also contains a cancer-fighting phytochemical called squalene. In addition to whisking it into salad dressings, try using olive oil as a healthier alternative to butter or margarine on your bread.

Another great oil is canola. It comes from a strain of rapeseed that Canadian agronomists bred specifically to improve its nutritional profile. In fact, the name "canola" is a combination of the words "Canadian" and "oil." More than 60 percent of its fatty acids are monounsaturates. The rest are mainly polyunsaturates—the essential omega-6 and omega-3 oils. Canola contains the highest ratio of omega-3s to omega-6s of any other oil you will eat regularly. That's important because thousands of years ago, the human diet contained a relatively balanced mix of these essential fatty acids. But today—because we eat so much omega-6-laden corn and cottonseed oil—we consume about 20 times more omega-6s than -3s. And that imbalance can lead to trouble. An excess of omega-6 oils can promote inflammation and blood clumping. The omega-3s, by contrast, reduce inflammation and are associated with lower levels of heart disease, hypertension, and diabetes. You need a good ratio, and you'll get it in canola oil.

If all of this sounds confusing, Dr. Artemis Simopoulos, an authority on essential fatty acids, has very simple advice: "Stop eating corn oil," she says. "Use olive or canola oil. Eat fish two or three times a week. That's all you need to remember."

Flip Over Flaxseed

Mahatma Gandhi once said, "Wherever flaxseeds become a regular food item among the people, there will be better health." Flaxseeds contain omega-3 oils, and they're a great source of dietary fiber, protein, iron, and potassium. In addition, they are by far the leading dietary source of a class of compounds called *lignans*, which are phytoestrogens, or plant estrogens. Like the indole-3-carbinol in broccoli, lignans alter the balance of estrogens in the body, favoring the production of an estrogen metabolite that appears to protect against breast cancer. Nutritionist Joanne Slavin at the University of Minnesota conducted two studies—one in premenopausal women and one in postmenopausal women—and found that in both groups, the balance of estrogens shifted in a favorable direction when the women ate a few tablespoons of flaxseed a day.

Flaxseeds can be purchased whole, cracked, or milled. The advantage to buying whole seeds is that the omega-3 fatty acids in them won't oxidize on your shelf, since the outer coating of the seeds shields the acids within. The drawback is that the human body is unable to digest the uncracked seeds, so you need to grind them in the coffee grinder before eating them. Dan Nadeau throws some into his smoothie in the morning and lets the blender do the work. Other ideas: Sprinkle the ground seeds on your cereal in the morning, or add them to bread or muffin dough the next time you bake. You can also add a spoonful of flaxseed oil to your smoothie.

Note: As wonderful as flaxseed is, it is important not to consume more than two to three tablespoons per day, because the husks contain compounds that can be toxic in high doses.

Munch a (Small) Bunch of Nuts

Sure, they're high in fat. That's why you shouldn't eat the whole bowl of peanuts at your next party. But most of the fats in nuts are the "good" kind. Walnuts in particular have high levels of omega-3 oils, not to mention cancer-fighting ellagic acid. Other types of nuts boast monounsaturated fats. And just about every type of nut is chock full of protein, fiber, potassium, magnesium, and vitamin E. "One Brazil nut gives you all the selenium you need for a day," says dietician Maureen Ternus, who is a consultant to the International Tree Nut Council's nutrition committee. Almonds are particularly high in riboflavin and vitamin E, pistachios in potassium and vitamin B_6, pine nuts in iron and thiamin, cashews in magnesium and copper. So go ahead, indulge. . . . in moderation. Nothing can jazz up a vegetable entrée like a handful of slivered almonds, toasted walnuts, or pine nuts.

Nuts also contain hefty amounts of cholesterol-lowering phytosterols. That may be one reason why clinical trials show that moderate nut intake reduces levels of "bad" cholesterol in the blood—and why major studies show that people who eat small amounts of nuts on a regular basis have dramatically lower levels of heart disease. The Nurses' Health Study found that women who ate about five ounces of nuts a week reduced their risk by 35 percent, compared to the non–nut-eaters. The Iowa Women's Health Study documented a 40 percent decrease in those who ate nuts just four times a month. And the Adventist Health Study found a 50 percent cut in those participants who consumed nuts five or more times a week. If you want a reason to eat nuts, that's it, in a nutshell.

Be a Mushroom Maven

Mushrooms aren't colorful. They're not even vegetables (they're fungi). But they're worth adding to your diet anyway. In the ancient world, people thought they were food for the gods—perhaps even born of thunder, since they appeared overnight after rainstorms. We agree that they're small miracles. Today scientists know that mushrooms are rich in many vitamins and minerals that are not abundant in other produce. The mineral selenium, which is thought to cut prostate cancer risk, is one. Copper is another. And mushrooms have significant amounts of three B-complex vitamins—riboflavin, niacin, and pantothenic acid.

THE SEVEN-DAY MEAL PLAN

You may still be thinking you can't possibly eat so many fruits, vegetables, whole grains, and legumes. But take a look at our seven-day meal plan. We obviously don't expect you to follow it to the letter. Rather, this sample plan gives you some ideas about how you can reach a daily goal of 100+ points.

Nutritionally, the seven-day meal plan is fit as a fiddle. You can rest assured that we've done all the major number crunching for you, so throw out your calculator and pocket calorie counter, and pick up your fork instead! Here's the skinny on the important "nutrition bites":

- **Total calories.** We have aimed for 2,000 calories a day, which the FDA considers to be an average daily requirement. For some of you, this may be too high—especially if you lead a sedentary life or are aiming for weight loss. For others, it may be too low. Feel free to adjust accordingly.
- **Percent of calories from fat.** Controlling your fat intake is an essential objective in any plan for optimum health. In our seven-day program an average of 25 percent of calories come from fat. (If your goal is weight loss, reduce that to 15 to 20 percent.) Remember that "good" fats are essential to the body, but that nearly all experts recommend keeping them below 30 percent of total calories.
- **Complex carbohydrates.** These are not "bad words" in the Color Code program. Complex or unrefined carbohydrates provide the key energy source for your brain and body—glucose. As numerous medical-school biochemistry textbooks say, "Fat burns in the fire of carbohydrates." To keep those fires burning, the percent of total calories from complex carbs should average 65 percent. Again, we've taken care of this for you.
- **Protein.** Most Americans are needlessly worried about getting sufficient protein. The seven-day plan with its focus on whole foods naturally supplies the requisite 10 to 15 percent of calories that should come from this source.
- **Cholesterol.** Your body can make all the cholesterol it needs, so aim to keep dietary cholesterol low. Except on Day 4 (which features an omelet), we provide about 50 milligrams a day, which is well below the American Heart Association's upper limit of 300.
- **Fiber.** Bulking up on fiber is one of the best things you can do for your body. The seven-day plan provides a healthy 50 grams a day—which is twice the daily value, or three to five times more than the average American eats.

NOTE: As you go through the plan, you'll see that the names of many dishes are capitalized. This means that the recipe for that dish appears in the recipe section of the book. Also, you'll notice that the basic color score, color bonus points, total color score, total calories, and percent of calories from fat appear at the end of each day's entry. (For beverage suggestions, see the section "Drink to Your Health" on page 184.) Bon appétit!

Day 1

Breakfast

Dan's Blueberry-Banana Smoothie; whole-wheat bagel with low-fat cream cheese

Snack

Orange

Lunch

Anne's West 57th Street Salad; multigrain bread

Snack

Popcorn with herb seasoning

Dinner

Blue corn chips and Chunky Guacamole; Baja Vegetable Stew; Spanish Rice; Kale with Garlic

Snack

Choice of blackberries, raspberries, or blueberries

Color Score:	120
Color Bonus Points:	60
Total Color Score:	180
Totals for Day 1: 1,922 calories; 30 percent of calories from fat	

Day 2

Breakfast

Low-fat yogurt topped with blueberries; orange juice; whole-wheat English muffin and natural peanut butter

Snack
   Apple

Lunch
   Sweet Pepper Vegetarian Chili; toasted whole wheat pita
   wedges

Snack
   Cantaloupe

Dinner
   Risotto by the Sea; Orange-Fennel Salad; crusty rye bread

Snack
   Strawberries and kiwifruit

Color Score:	100
Color Bonus Points:	45
Total Color Score:	145
Totals for Day 2: 2,118 calories; 20 percent of calories from fat	

Day 3

Breakfast
   Banana raisin oatmeal; fresh orange sections

Snack
   Cantaloupe

Lunch
   Veggie burger on whole-wheat bread or bun; Southwestern
   Rice Salad

Snack
   Fresh cherries

Dinner
   Jim's Salmon Sergio; brown rice; Red and Green Beans with
   Pine Nuts

Snack
   Blueberries with (optional) lemon yogurt topping

Color Score: 70
Color Bonus Points: 30
Total Color Score: 100
Totals for Day 3: 1,950 calories; 23 percent of calories from fat

Day 4

Breakfast
Orange juice; Free-Range Confetti Omelet; pumpernickel toast with almond butter

Snack
Red grapes

Lunch
Colorful Vegetable Fajitas; Tabouli

Snack
Mixed nuts

Dinner
Shiitake Mushroom Miso Soup; two California Rolls with Sushi Rice

Snack
Blueberries

Color Score: 80
Color Bonus Points: 45
Total Color Score: 125
Totals for Day 4: 2,133 calories; 32 percent of calories from fat

Day 5

Breakfast
Low-fat granola with low-fat or soy milk and raspberries

Snack
Fresh grapefruit sections

Lunch
  Brazilian Black Bean Soup; Skillet Cornbread

Snack
  Raisins

Dinner
  Haddock with Olive Oil and Garlic; Royal Basmati Rice;
  Spinach Salad with Tarragon Vinegar and Toasted Almonds

Snack
  Blueberry-Granola Bars

Color Score:	90
Color Bonus Points:	40
Total Color Score:	130
Totals for Day 5: 2,110 calories; 20 percent of calories from fat	

Day 6

Breakfast
  Roasted Potatoes with Red Pepper and Onion; veggie sausage

Snack
  Banana

Lunch
  Gypsy Soup; multigrain bread

Snack
  Plum

Dinner
  Grilled Free-Range Chicken Breasts; Rosemary Roasted Sweet
  Potatoes; Sesame Kale

Snack
  Cut-up peaches and blueberries

Color Score: 110
Color Bonus: 40
Total Color Score: 150
Totals for Day 6: 1,803 calories; 29 percent of calories from fat

Day 7

Breakfast
Buckwheat Banana Pancakes with Blueberry Sauce; Paradise Freeze

Snack
Pear

Lunch
Gingered Carrot Soup; Chickpea Basil Spread with Pita Chips

Snack
Kiwifruit

Dinner
Curried Eggplant with Spinach over brown rice; whole wheat French bread

Snack
Mango Smoothie

Color Score: 100
Color Bonus Points: 45
Total Color Score: 145
Totals for Day 7: 1,945 calories, 23 percent of calories from fat

THE FAST-FOOD DIET: A REALITY CHECK
"Americans are digging their graves with their knives and forks," wrote Dr. Joel Fuhrman in *Fasting and Eating for Health*. Never was this more true than today. With its fast food and sodas, the standard American diet (appropriately abbreviated as SAD) packs

in the calories and fat. At the same time, it skimps on colorful fruits and vegetables. Mary Fleming, the dietician who provided the nutritional analysis of our seven-day diet plan, says that a typical diet for many of her patients looks something like this:

Breakfast
   Egg and sausage on a biscuit
   Hash browns
   Coffee with cream and sugar

Lunch
   Cheeseburger with bacon
   French fries
   Vanilla shake

Dinner
   Fried chicken
   Mashed potatoes with gravy
   Cole slaw
   Soda
   Ice cream

Do you wonder how this regimen stacks up against the Color Code meal plan? Here's the bad news. This typical SAD day packs 3,560 calories—and that's using normal serving sizes, with no second helpings or between-meal treats. A whopping 53 percent of those calories come from fat. Cholesterol tops the charts at 850 milligrams. And fiber is just 28 percent of the recommended daily level. On a typical Color Code day by contrast, calories average 2,000. Fat is just 25 percent, with a mere 50 milligrams of cholesterol. And fiber is double the daily value. As you can tell at a glance, the SAD day also falls short on color. No wonder Dan Nadeau refers to the standard American diet as a "flatliner diet."

ACTION STARTERS

A scoring system and a seven-day meal plan are a good start. We've also tried to provide tips on how to make your meals more colorful. But if you're not already eating this way, chances are you still need a little more help turning thought to action. After all, it's hard to break lifelong habits. Here are several practical suggestions to help you start eating more colorfully.

Keep a Color Counter

This is a good way to get a sense of how high your color score really is—and how far you have to go. Start with a fresh piece of paper and write four headings on it—Red, Orange-Yellow, Green, and Blue-Purple. Every time you eat a serving of fruits or vegetables, jot it down under the appropriate heading. Write everything down as soon as you've eaten it, because people tend to eat more food than they realize—and quickly forget what they've eaten. At the end of the day, go through the list and add up your color score, being sure to give yourself credit for bonus points. If you are like many Americans, you may score between 25 and 50. Don't be discouraged! This is your opportunity to look over the list and see where you could have done better. You have to start somewhere.

Use the Replacement Method

Believe us, we know how hard it is to break old habits. And we also know that different people need different strategies to get started on a major change in the way they eat. The replacement method works for some folks. If you stick with it, it will take about two weeks from the time you start to the time you're ready to use the whole-day suggestions in the seven-day plan.

Here's how it works: on day one, replace *one* dessert or snack with a serving of fruit. Done. Now, that wasn't so bad. On day two (or at a comfortable interval), replace two items—for example, one snack and your breakfast choice—with two items that reflect the Color Code eating principles. On day three, replace three items—perhaps a snack, a breakfast item, and one side dish at dinner. The really big changes will come when you stop tinkering around the edges and replace main courses with fabulous veggie entrées. The goal is not to deprive yourself of good food, but to make healthy food that tastes great.

It helps to keep a log (or the back of a blank envelope shoved in your back pocket—whatever's easy for you) to track how you're doing each day. By the end of two weeks, you're to be eating the Color Code way—and feeling very proud of yourself, too.

Banish the Trans Fats

Did you ever wonder about the partially hydrogenated vegetable oils that seem to crop up in almost every processed food? Wonder no more. Avoid them. You might as well be eating lard.

The process of hydrogenation turns a nice liquid vegetable oil into an unhealthy solid fat known as a "trans fat." In the process, it also destroys essential fatty acids—the omega-3s and omega-6s that your body cannot make for itself. Manufacturers like to use trans fats for two reasons. First, these fats are resistant to oxidation, so products keep well on store shelves. Second, they provide the texture of butter, but allow manufacturers to print the healthy-sounding words "vegetable oil" on the product label rather than the not-so-healthy-sounding "butter."

Don't be taken in. Authorities say that trans fats actually are the most harmful of all the fats. Like saturated fats, they raise "bad" cholesterol. But they're even worse than saturated fats, because they also lower "good" cholesterol. That's bad news, because Americans eat a lot of trans fats. Just about every package of cookies, crackers, candy, donuts, chips, biscuits, muffins, and pastries on the market contains these fats. Think of it as one more reason to snack on fruit instead.

By the way, sometime in the next two years, a listing for trans fats will start appearing in the "Nutrition Facts" boxes on food labels. Watch for it!

Change Your Mental Image of Dinner

If you ask people on the street what they're having for dinner, chances are the answer will be "beef," "pork," or some other type of meat. In essence, they're building a meal around a dead animal—a food without color points, at that. But here's an idea. Try answering the question "What's for dinner?" with the response "Wild rice and vegetables." That sounds strange at first. But it doesn't mean that you have to limit dinner to plain boiled rice and steamed broccoli. The recipe section at the back of the book includes vegetable fajitas, eggplant-spinach curry, and watercress salad with pears, among many other delicious entrées.

As fruits and vegetables move to the center of your plate, meat will inevitably move to the edges or off altogether. Ideally, you will start to think of meat as a side dish. That's what the Chinese do. It's also one reason why the Chinese are comparatively so healthy. The traditional Chinese way of conceptualizing a meal is known as *fan tsai*. *Fan* means "rice"—but in the larger scheme of things, it can also stand for noodles, sorghum, steamed bread, or another staple that forms the core of the meal. It is the starch at the center of the plate. *Tsai* literally means "vegetables," but it can also stand for whatever you add to the staple. "It is most likely to be vegetables," says Nina Simonds, author of an Asian-style cookbook called *A Spoonful of Ginger*. "But the Chinese also eat a little seafood. They rarely eat meat."

Simonds learned about Asian cooking when she moved to Taiwan at the age of 19 and settled in with a Chinese family. Meals there consisted of an individual bowl of rice for everyone, plus a variety of vegetarian or seafood dishes in the center of the table that one could use to garnish the rice. Simonds, however, objected to eating so much rice. "Like other American teenagers, I thought rice was fattening, so I'd ask for just half a bowl of rice and focus on foods in the center of the table," says Simonds. "My surrogate Chinese family soon started calling me *da pigu*, which means the 'big pig,' because I was filling my bowl with what were supposed to be the garnishes." Now in her 40s, Simonds has long since overhauled her eating habits and put the garnishes back on the side. She's also become a best-selling cookbook author.

How to Dine Out Colorfully

You may already be changing your mental image of dinner. But unfortunately, most restaurant owners are not. As a result, finding color-rich meals in restaurants is often challenging. Here are a few simple strategies that will help.

- Start with fruit juice instead of soda. Cranberry juice or orange juice will earn you color points.
- Order side dishes of vegetables.
- Request fruit for dessert. Most good restaurants will have fresh berries. If you don't see them on the menu, ask. Dan Nadeau does this all the time.

Find Recipes That Can Earn You Major Points

That's not hard to do, if you glance through the recipe section in this book. Dan's Blueberry-Banana Smoothie is a two-serving drink that will earn you 25 points (10 apiece for two servings of fruit and a 5-point bonus for making one of them blueberries). Baja Vegetable Stew counts as 2.5 servings. Our Gazpacho with Fresh Herbs counts as 3 servings. If you remember how small a serving of vegetables really is, you'll see how easy it is to accumulate servings—and points!

Find Seven Color-Filled Recipes and Learn Them by Heart

As much as we encourage variety, we know that people tend to eat the same foods over and over. This is just reality, especially today, when so many couples work outside the home. Who has the energy to toil in the office for eight hours, then get out the recipe books and experiment with new ingredients? The key is to learn a few really healthy recipes that you love and can use as fallbacks when you're too weary to experiment. (Keeping them posted on the fridge can help, while you're still learning the recipes.) Cardiologist William Castelli, former head of the Framingham Heart Study, has said that Americans could largely eliminate heart disease if everyone would simply adopt ten new healthy recipes.

Develop a Crush on Garlic

Some of those new recipes should include garlic. Jim Joseph adds it to almost every main course he cooks, and for good reason. For thousands of years, garlic has had a vast store of medicinal uses. The ancient Greek physician Dioscorides reported that garlic could "clear the arteries," and Hippocrates prescribed it for intestinal disorders. In 1858, Louis Pasteur discovered that garlic could kill bacteria. And because Russian physicians used the garlic bulb to cure infections it was known as "Russian penicillin" well into the 20th century. Albert Schweitzer is even said to have used garlic as a cure for amoebic dysentery when he was in Africa.

With thousands of years of folk medicine behind it, garlic is now proving to be a star in lab tests as well. Scientists have identified more than 200 compounds in it, including at least 20 germ killers. Garlic also contains numerous antioxidants and more than a dozen anti-inflammatories. But the garlic compounds that are gaining the most attention are the organosulfur compounds, which are similar to those found in onions, leeks, and chives. They are thought to be responsible for garlic's antibacterial and antifungal activities, as well its ability to slow cholesterol synthesis, lower blood pressure, reduce atherosclerosis, and inhibit platelet aggregation. The sulfur compounds may even prove to fight cancer. In the Iowa Women's Health Study, women who ate garlic at least once a week had a 32 percent lower risk of colon cancer than those who ate none. Research at the National Cancer Institute is showing that garlic extracts can both slow the proliferation of cancer cells and cause abnormal cells to self-destruct.

John Milner, professor of nutrition at Pennsylvania State University and acting chief of the nutrition science research group at the National Cancer Institute, says the secret to getting the most benefit out of garlic is to chop the cloves and let them sit for 10 to 15 minutes. That's because the organosulfur compounds do not form until you've sliced into the bulb. He also suggests eating garlic together with selenium-rich foods, such as fish and whole grains, since selenium appears to increase garlic's efficacy. "Selenium works with garlic to block the formation of compounds associated with cancer initiation and cell proliferation," says Milner.

Pressed for Time? Rediscover Soups, Salads, and Fruit to Go

Nothing packs a walloping color score like a vegetable soup or fresh tossed salad. When you have the time, spend a leisurely weekend afternoon making a wonderful soup or chili that's chock full of vegetables. It's relaxing—even therapeutic—fills the house with wonderful aromas, and results in as many as three meals to get you through the beginning of the week. However, we also know that once the week kicks in, it can be hard to find time for cooking. So if you're in a pinch, remember that soups—and salads, too—are easy to pick up at the prepared foods counter at your local supermarket, deli, or gourmet takeout. Presliced fruit can save you time as well.

Keep an Emergency Stash in Your Pantry, Purse, Desk Drawer, and Glove Compartment

Nothing derails you faster than not having healthy food handy when your stomach is grumbling and you're on the run. What if you don't have time to cook a proper dinner before your parent-teacher conference or your child's basketball game? You won't have to worry if you stock your pantry and freezer with items like canned vegetable soup and frozen berries for fast smoothies. What if you're stuck in a traffic jam? Reach in your glove compartment and open that zippered plastic bag of dried apricots. Logjam in the doctor's waiting room? Plan ahead and pick up a can of V8 or an apple on the way.

One of the worst places for snack attacks is the office. When they strike, don't sneak off to the vending machine. Get in the habit of bringing fresh fruit to work every day. Or keep a space in your desk drawer for healthy "grab it" items like boxes of raisins, packs of cashews, or dried cranberries. You get the idea. Be creative! And remember, variety is the key to offsetting boredom. Change the contents of your "grab it" spots on a regular basis.

Grow a Vegetable Garden

There is an incomparable sense of wonder that comes from watching your own vegetables grow. For many people, growing a garden may not be possible. But even if you live in a crowded city, a small patch of earth or a community garden are places where you can plant a packet of tomato seeds. Aside from the satisfaction of watching your vegetables come up, there are two reasons why doing this will help you increase your color score:

- Food just tastes better when it's fresh-picked. Nothing is as divine as fresh basil and dill. Tomatoes are redder and juicier when allowed to ripen on the vine. All this positive reinforcement will encourage you to eat fresh produce.
- When a crop ripens, you will probably have a lot of it—and that forces you to get creative with new recipes. Zucchini, for example, almost always yields a bumper crop. Suddenly you're inspired to find a dozen new ways to use the squash—in zucchini soup, zucchini bread, zucchini lasagna, ratatouille, and so on. The more tasty recipes you find for zucchini, the more likely you are to cook with it in the future.

Be Kind to the Earth: Buy Organic

Since 1945, insecticide use in this country has increased tenfold. The implications are pretty scary. But does this mean you should avoid fruits and vegetables? Hardly. By simply washing them thoroughly with warm water, you can eliminate most of the pesticide residues on the skins. Of course, that won't help you get rid of pesticides *inside* the fruit. (Plants can suck up noxious chemicals along with water from the soil.) But on balance, the benefits of cancer-fighting phytochemicals far outweigh the minimal risks of pesticide residues.

That said, there is a better way still. Eat organic produce, if you can. It may be more expensive, but you can often find better prices at farmers markets, coops, buying clubs, and community supported farms. Not only is organic produce safer for your family, but it's also kinder and gentler on the environment. Agriculture is a major polluter of American rivers and streams. Organic farming, however, does not contaminate our water. Soil that is farmed organically becomes richer from year to year, rather than being depleted over time. That makes for more sustainable farming—and sustainability will become especially important over the next 50 years, as the world population grows by an estimated three billion. "Organic food not only stands for a healthier you, but also a healthier planet," says Andrew Kimbrell, director of the Center for Food Safety in Washington, D.C.

THE TRUTH IN BLACK
AND WHITE

"Our lives are not in the lap of the gods, but in the lap of
our cooks."
—Lin Yutang, *The Importance of Living* (1937)

ON A CONCEPTUAL LEVEL AT LEAST, black and white—reflecting no colors and all colors—also have their uses. Together, they give us the sense that we can see the world in clear-cut terms. Like yin and yang, they tug at each other, balancing each other out, letting us delineate differences between one thing and another. As long as we can grasp an issue in black and white, we know where we stand.

Unfortunately, when it comes to nutrition, black and white seem to switch places with disconcerting regularity. First we were supposed to avoid butter; then the experts announced that margarine was even worse. For years, we tried to eliminate fat; then carbohydrates became the focus of our concerns. Caffeine seems to go through more ups and downs than hemlines. No wonder people are confused.

When it comes to individual phytonutrients, the scientific wisdom will also inevitably change. New studies will continue to pour in from labs around the country. Some of them may contradict one or another of the findings here. But even if they do, this book will be timeless. Here's why.

DISCOVERING BLACK AND WHITE

There is one absolute black-and-white truth—a single principle that forms the solid bedrock of this book. This truth is that a low-fat diet based on fruits, vegetables, and whole grains offers the best possible diet for achieving optimum health. "God has done the randomized, controlled trial," declares Dr. David Heber, professor of medicine and director of the UCLA Center for Human Nutrition. And the results of that trial show that populations around the world who eat in this manner, exercise regularly, and avoid tobacco have the fewest occurrences of cancer, heart disease, hypertension, diabetes, and osteoporosis.

That's why you don't need to fret over the latest headlines. Don't sweat the small stuff. If you stick to the principles we've outlined here—think color, think variety, think whole foods— you'll do fine. It's a simple approach that anyone can use. It's scientifically sound. What's more, it's fun. You don't have to count calories or get bogged down in buying large quantities of quercetin supplements or indole-3-carbinol pills. In fact, the opposite is true. "People always want to isolate a chemical and put it in a pill," says nutritionist Susan Davis of Damariscotta, Maine. "Well, now we know that *food* is the magic bullet."

In this book, we've presented the latest findings about phytochemicals not so that you will rush out and buy lycopene supplements, but so that you'll eat tomatoes. We hope you will skip the bottled extracts and reach instead for crisp spinach and juicy blueberries. This is what dieticians mean when they refer to the "new nutrition"—relying not on pills, but on food, to meet our nutritional needs. And these professionals reserve special praise for the most colorful, deeply pigmented, gloriously vibrant fruits and vegetables.

Some people may secretly hope that this framework will be overturned by later research, like those other flimsy dictums that were so easily reversed. Don't count on it. We're in black-and-white territory here. As health columnist Jane E. Brody put it in the *New York Times*: "Cached away in the soul of every red-blooded American who fondly recalls when carnivory was a virtue, and supper wasn't supper without a centerpiece of pork chops or prime rib, lies the frail hope that all the recent emphasis on fruits, grains, and vegetables, vegetables, vegetables, will somehow turn out to be a terrible mistake. Well, abandon that hope, ye who harbor it."

FAT-FREE NONSENSE

The bulk of a healthy diet should come from the foods we've discussed in this book—fruits, vegetables, legumes, whole grains, fish, tea, juices, and nuts. That may sound perfectly obvious. But with so much conflicting information out there, confusion still reigns. Dan Nadeau sees patients every day who think they're eating well just because they're avoiding red meat. In fact, their diets are often deplorable. A teenage girl may avoid hamburgers, but subsist on iceberg lettuce and Coke. A busy lawyer may cut out filet mignon, but fill up on cheese, pizza, and donuts. In either of these regimens, where are the protective phytochemicals? Are these folks getting anywhere close to the 25 grams of fiber they need to consume in a day? Are they eating from every color group? Of course not.

Not only do these common ways of eating provide little nutrition, but they also lack built-in mechanisms of portion control. When you dine on a baked potato, you're likely to stop after one. Total calories: 100. When you rip open a large bag of chips, you can easily eat half the bag—and occasionally polish off a whole one. Total calories: 700 or so.

Other people load up on fat-free baked goods and think they're doing their bodies a favor. If so, then why has the national girth expanded since the introduction of fat-free cookies, cakes, brownies, and ice cream? It turns out that many fat-free foods compensate for the loss of fat by adding high-fructose corn syrup and other empty calories. Reducing fat is not a goal in itself, if all you do is bulk up on junk food—even if it is fat-free junk food.

Fortunately, the public has come to realize that fat-free brownies will save neither our health nor our waistlines. Now it's time to start reeducating the public about carbohydrates, too.

CARBOHYDRATES: NO FEAR

Just as fear of fat swept the nation a decade ago, fear of carbohydrates is seizing the public today. Certain diet programs have demonized carbohydrates, and the anti-carb message has filtered through to just about every fitness magazine you pick up. But the problem with the standard American diet isn't that it includes a lot of carbohydrates. It's the type of carbs that constitutes the problem—soft drinks, cakes, cookies, chips, and so forth. In short, junk food. The rap on carbohydrates is that they'll make you fat. Well, sure they will plump you up, if you're bingeing on junk food. But carbohydrates also include nourishing whole grains and low-calorie fruits and vegetables. To their credit, many of the anti-carb crowd draw this vital distinction. To the extent that they've helped steer people away from candy bars and sodas, they've performed a real service.

Unfortunately, the anti-carb crusaders have also spread a number of half-truths. These folks explain (correctly) that the body converts carbohydrates into glucose. As glucose enters the bloodstream, the body responds by releasing insulin, which enables your muscles and organs to absorb the glucose. So far, so good. But these sources go astray when they say that insulin also readily converts extra glucose to fat. Not so. In fact, your body does everything it can to keep glucose reserves in tight balance and will increase its metabolism to prevent too much glucose from being stored. Only tiny amounts—two to four grams a day—can be put away as fat, even with extremely high carb intake. By contrast, the body can store dietary fats in unlimited quantities—and gram for gram, fats have more than twice as many calories as carbohydrates. Why, then, do people lose weight on low-carb diets? Not because they're lowering their insulin levels, but because they're actually reducing their caloric intake.

Some books and magazine articles take the anti-carb argument one step further. They say that carbohydrates are digested quickly, provoking dangerous spikes in insulin that can exacerbate diabetes and even possibly contribute to the development of the disease. But the carbohydrates that rush into the bloodstream quickly are mainly processed foods made from refined sugar and flour—not whole grains such as buckwheat, vegetables like carrots and sweet potatoes, or even sweet fruits like cherries and dried apricots. Refined sugar and flour behave differently because they have been pulverized into fine granules that the body does not have to work hard to digest—and because they are conspicuously lacking in fiber. As you know by now, fiber slows the release of sugar into the bloodstream, like a timed-release capsule. Refined foods aren't the carbs you want to eat anyway. As we've been saying, many of them are no better than junk food. "Eating white bread is very much like eating plain sugar, as far as your body knows," says Walter Willett, chairman of nutrition at Harvard's School of Public Health.

IN PRAISE OF CARBOHYDRATES

Whole grains are a different matter entirely. They are rich in vitamins, minerals, and fiber—and they are definitely part of a healthy diet. Every major civilization from Asia to the Americas has had grain as a staple. Wheat is said to have been the world's most important crop since it originated in western Asia around 8,000 B.C. Rice, too, has been a sustainer of Asian civilizations—just like millet in northern Africa, oats in Scotland, and corn in the Americas. From Italy to China, grain products like pasta and noodles have been central to numerous cuisines. Recently, people have rediscovered quinoa, the ancient grain of the Incas, and the highly nutritious "supergrain" called amaranth. Throughout the ages, people have consumed these grains in minimally processed forms that preserve their health benefits.

Indeed, the fact that these grains could be stored from one season to the next historically allowed people to end the nomadic life and begin developing systems of writing, mathematics, science, and art—in short, civilization. While humans are omnivorous, the ideal diet takes this lesson from history and recognizes that grain is a key to healthy nutrition. So is that other great source of carbohydrates—fresh produce.

These are precisely the carbohydrates you want to eat—whole grains, fruits, and vegetables.

FROM BLACK-AND-WHITE TO LIVING COLOR

A number of diets already fit this health-promoting formula. The Mediterranean diet is one. It's rich in olive oil, fresh fruits, vegetables, fish, nuts, and beans. The traditional Japanese diet is another healthy choice. It includes a lot of rice, fish, soy, green tea, and a large range of colorful fresh vegetables.

Whatever eating regimen you choose, the guiding principle is that you need to paint your color palette every day with red, orange, green, and blue. Colorful foods—fruits and vegetables across the spectrum—help protect you against the worst ravages of old age. In many ways, they're the most powerful medicine we have available.

Lately, so much political debate has focused on prescription drug coverage. But think about this a minute. By changing what you eat, you can reduce your blood pressure, lower your blood sugar, and diminish the risks of cancer, heart disease, and macular degeneration. You can do all these things without pricey pharmaceuticals, just by adopting a more healthy, semi-vegetarian diet— one loaded with dark, leafy greens, deep orange vegetables, and vibrant red and blue fruits. No politician ever mentions this, of course. Healthy eating is not a platform that would get a person elected to any office, except president of the food co-op. But you can do all these good things for yourself just by eating a colorful diet. As a Greek adage says, "It is the function of medicine to help people die young as late as possible." Food is precisely the medicine that lets you do that. Colorful food, that is.

A joke circulating on the Internet purports to relate the history of medicine.

> *2000 B.C.—Here, eat this root.*
> *1000 B.C.—That root is heathen. Here, say this prayer.*
> *A.D. 1850—That prayer is superstition. Here, drink his potion.*
> *A.D. 1940—That potion is snake oil. Here, swallow this pill.*
> *A.D. 1985—That pill is ineffective. Here, take this antibiotic.*
> *A.D. 2000—That antibiotic doesn't work anymore. Here, eat this root.*

The only thing we would add is to make sure that root is colorful. It may be the best medicine available.

THE COLOR CODE RECIPES

E VEN WITH ALL THE SUGGESTIONS presented in this book, it can still be challenging to eat 10 or more servings of fruits and vegetables a day. Many people ask, "How can I integrate these servings into my regular meal routine? If I have to eat more fruits and vegetables, then that means I have to eat even more food. How can it work?"

When you incorporate more fruits and vegetables into your diet, you naturally eliminate other foods that are less healthy and nutrient-dense. These recipes are designed to help you replace empty-calorie food choices with healthy choices and to inspire you to try new fruits and vegetables, like mangoes or kale, that you may not have tried before because you don't know what to make with them.

In addition to helping you eat more produce servings a day, the recipes are designed with one top priority in mind: great flavor and irresistible combinations of fruits and vegetables, along with pasta, meat, poultry, and fish and seafood. All the recipes contain at least one serving of fruits or vegetables and most contain two or even three fruit or vegetable servings. Look for soups, salads, and smoothies to get the most bang for your buck.

Since it can sometimes be hard, even impossible, to prepare breakfast, lunch, and dinner in your kitchen, try instead to target one meal a day, such as a weeknight dinner or a leisurely weekend lunch, to pack several servings into one meal. Here are just a few to get you started:

- Paradise Freeze, 2.5 servings (page 291)
- Dan's Blueberry-Banana Smoothie, 2 servings (page 290)

- Five-Fruit Salad, 2.5 servings (page 234)
- Zucchini, Red Pepper, and Leek Frittata: 2.5 servings (page 287)
- Jim's Salmon Sergio, 2 servings (page 260)
- Artichoke and Roasted Red Pepper Salad with Roasted Red Pepper Dressing, 2.5 servings (page 238)
- Sweet Potato Black Bean Salad, 2.5 servings (page 245)
- Anne's West 57th Street Salad, 2 servings (page 237)
- Spring Greens and Polenta Pie, 2 servings (page 282)
- Gazpacho with Fresh Herbs, 3 servings (page 229)
- Sweet Pepper Vegetarian Chili, 2.5 servings (page 256)
- Baja Vegetable Stew, 2.5 servings (page 253)
- Brazilian Black Bean Soup, 2 servings (page 227)
- Gypsy Soup, 2 servings (page 231)

We encourage you to mix and match recipes to create your daily menus. See how easy it is to rack up servings fast—have a soup made with two vegetables and a cup of fruit salad for dessert and you've just knocked off four or five servings in one sitting! The point is to have fun and to see just how delicious your meals can be—with the extra bonus of increasing your intake of fruits and vegetables. You're certain to learn some great new ways to create meals, such as smoothies for breakfast and dishes where vegetables, not meat, take center stage. Keep yourself challenged to discover new favorites and combinations.

As you plan your weekly shopping, choose a handful of recipes to try, and purchase the ingredients you need ahead of time. That always saves time in the kitchen. After familiarizing yourself with the recipes here, you may just find yourself creating your own Color Code recipes!

Appetizers, Salsas, and Soups	
Chickpea with Basil Spread	222
Hummus Dip with Toasted Sesame	223
Chunky Guacamole	224
Tabouli	224

Side Dishes

APPETIZERS, SALSAS, AND SOUPS

Chickpea with Basil Spread

8 tablespoons low-sodium, light
    mayonnaise
4 tablespoons chopped fresh basil
2 tablespoons sun-dried tomatoes

1 teaspoon fresh lemon juice
¼ teaspoon freshly ground pepper
1 can (15 ounces) chickpeas or
    garbanzo beans

In a food processor, combine all the ingredients and process until smooth. Transfer the mixture to a medium-size bowl and chill in the refrigerator.

Serves 8.
Nutritional analysis, per serving: calories, 91; fat, 3g; cholesterol, 5mg; carbohydrate, 14g; fiber, 3g; protein, 3g; calories from fat, 4%

Used with permission from the Ellsworth Cooking School, Ellsworth, Maine.

Hummus Dip with Toasted Sesame

1 can (20 ounces) garbanzo beans

2 cloves garlic, minced

¼ cup lemon juice

2 tablespoons toasted sesame

½ teaspoon ground cumin

½ teaspoon sesame oil

¼ teaspoon ground red pepper

1 tablespoon finely minced scallions

2 tablespoons chopped fresh
    parsley

Drain beans, reserving 2 tablespoons liquid. In a medium-size bowl, mash beans well with a potato masher (or use a food processor). Add the rest of the ingredients and mix well. If dip looks too dry, add liquid reserved from beans. Cover and chill at least 2 hours. Serve dip with crackers, breadsticks, or raw vegetables.

Makes 1¾ cups.
Nutritional analysis, per serving: calories, 31; fat, 8g; carbohydrate, 5g; fiber, 1g; protein, 2g; calories from fat, 2%

Used with permission from the Ellsworth Cooking School, Ellsworth, Maine.

Chunky Guacamole

••

2 tablespoons fresh lime juice or
  lemon juice
2 avocados
2 cloves garlic, minced
½ teaspoon salt
½ teaspoon ground cumin seed

½ teaspoon chili powder
⅛ teaspoon freshly ground pepper
⅛ teaspoon cayenne pepper
3 tablespoons low-calorie
  mayonnaise

In a medium bowl, add the lime juice and avocados (cut open the avocados, spoon out the flesh, and mash it with a fork until it's the desired consistency). Stir in the remaining ingredients; cover tightly and chill in the refrigerator.

Serves 8.
Nutritional analysis, per serving: calories, 97; fat, 9g; cholesterol, 1mg; carbohydrate, 5g; fiber, 2g; protein, 1g; calories from fat, 14%

Used with permission from the Ellsworth Cooking School, Ellsworth, Maine.

Tabouli

••

3 cups water
½ teaspoon salt
1 cup bulgur wheat
3 medium-size whole tomatoes,
  chopped
1 clove garlic, minced

4 tablespoons fresh chives
½ cup chopped fresh parsley
10 fresh peppermint leaves
8 tablespoons small white beans
2 tablespoons olive oil
4 tablespoons fresh lemon juice

In a large pot, boil water with salt. Once the water boils, add the bulgur. Let water return to a boil and then remove from heat. Keep covered for 20 minutes and drain any water left at the time. Chill in the refrigerator, stirring occasionally, until the bulgur cools. Add all the other ingredients. You can purée the tomatoes, chives, parsley, and mint together. Serve well chilled.

Makes 2 to 3 cups.
Nutritional analysis, per serving: calories, 150; fat, 4g; cholesterol, 0mg; carbohydrate, 26g; fiber, 7g; protein, 5g; calories from fat, 6%

Used with permission from the Ellsworth Cooking School, Ellsworth, Maine.

California Kiwifruit Salsa
. . . .

1½ cups (3 to 4) kiwifruit, peeled and diced

2 medium-size tangerines or 1 orange, peeled and diced

1 cup jicama, peeled and diced

½ cup red or yellow bell pepper, diced

½ to 1 small jalapeño pepper, minced, seeds and veins removed

¼ cup cilantro, chopped

1 tablespoon lime juice

1 tablespoon vegetable oil

¼ teaspoon salt

In a large bowl, combine all ingredients, mixing well. Chill briefly in the refrigerator before serving.

Makes 2½ cups.
Nutritional analysis, per serving: calories, 138; fat, 3g; carbohydrate, 15g; fiber, 4g; protein, 1g; calories from fat, 20%

Used with permission from the California Kiwifruit Commission.

Calypso Strawberry-Mango Salsa

• •

1 basket (12 ounces) of
strawberries, stemmed and
chopped
1 large mango, peeled, seeded, and
chopped
¼ cup green onion with tops, sliced

2 tablespoons fresh lime juice
1 tablespoon cilantro, chopped
½ teaspoon red pepper flakes
¼ teaspoon ground cumin
Salt, to taste

In a medium-size bowl, combine the strawberries, mango, onion, lime juice, cilantro, red pepper, and ground cumin. Mix in the salt. Serve immediately or cover the salsa and refrigerate up to two days. Serve the salsa with corn chips, chicken, or a mild white fish.

Makes 3 cups.
Nutritional analysis, per serving: calories, 22; fat, 0g; cholesterol, 0mg; carbohydrate, 6g; fiber, 1g; protein, 0g; calories from fat, 0%

Used with permission from the California Strawberry Commission.

Brazilian Black Bean Soup

••

2 cups dry black beans
3½ cups water or stock
2 teaspoons salt
2 tablespoons oil, approximately
1 cup chopped onion
3 cloves crushed garlic
1 large chopped carrot
1 stalk chopped celery
1 cup chopped green pepper, optional

1 teaspoon ground coriander
1½ teaspoons ground cumin
2 oranges, peeled, sectioned, and seeded
½ cup orange juice
1 tablespoon dry sherry
¼ teaspoon black pepper
¼ teaspoon red pepper
½ teaspoon fresh lemon juice

1. Rinse the beans. Cover them with water and let them soak at least 4 hours. Pour off the water. Place in a saucepan with 3½ cups water or stock and salt. Bring to a boil, cover, and simmer 1½ hours over very low heat.
2. Heat the oil in a skillet and cook the onions, garlic, carrot, celery, green pepper, coriander, and cumin. If necessary, add a little water to the vegetables to steam them along. When the mixture is finished cooking, add it to the beans. Let the soup continue to simmer over lowest possible heat.
3. Add the oranges, orange juice, sherry, black pepper, red pepper, and lemon juice to the soup. Stir the soup, cover, and sit down for 10 minutes. Now return to the soup, refreshed. Look at it and ask yourself if this soup suits you. Is it too thick? Add water. Do you want it thicker, heartier? You can puree some of it in a blender. You can make it hotter with more red pepper. Top with sour cream or yogurt.

Serves 5 to 6.
Nutritional analysis, per serving: calories, 330; fat, 6g; cholesterol, 0mg; carbohydrate, 55g; fiber, 13g; protein, 16g; calories from fat, 9%

Fusion Spiced Sweet Potato Soup

••

2 tablespoons butter

2 tablespoons finely grated fresh ginger

3 celery stalks, finely chopped (about 1 cup)

1 large onion, finely chopped (about 2 cups)

1 tablespoon curry powder

½ teaspoon cinnamon

¼ teaspoon cayenne pepper

⅛ teaspoon nutmeg

2½ pounds sweet potatoes, peeled and cut into ½-inch cubes

6 cups reduced-sodium chicken broth

½ teaspoon dried thyme

1 small bay leaf

¾ teaspoon salt

½ teaspoon pepper

½ cup milk

Sour cream for garnish

Chopped roasted peanuts for garnish

1. In a large pot, melt the butter over medium heat. Add ginger, celery, and onion, cook 5 to 7 minutes until soft. Add curry powder, cinnamon, cayenne, and nutmeg. Cook 1 minute, stirring constantly. Add sweet potatoes, broth, thyme, bay leaf, salt, and pepper. Increase heat to high and bring to a boil. Lower heat to medium and simmer 25 minutes or until the potatoes are soft and cooked through.

2. Transfer the soup in batches to a blender or food processor and puree. Thin the soup with milk. Garnish with a dollop of sour cream and some chopped peanuts.

Serves 12.
Nutritional analysis, per serving: calories, 179; fat, 4g; cholesterol, 8mg; carbohydrate, 28g; fiber, 4g; protein, 8g; calories from fat, 20%

Used with permission from the North Carolina SweetPotato Commission.

Gazpacho with Fresh Herbs

....

6 large tomatoes

1 large cucumber, peeled, seeded, and finely chopped

1 large green bell pepper, finely chopped

1 medium-size red onion, minced

3 tablespoons red wine vinegar

Juice of ½ lemon

2 tablespoons olive oil

2 to 3 tablespoons chopped fresh parsley

2 tablespoons chopped fresh basil

2 teaspoons salt and freshly ground pepper, to taste

Tabasco sauce, to taste

Herb croutons for garnish

1. Peel the tomatoes by submerging them in boiling water for 15 seconds. Remove to a colander and rinse under cold water. The skins should slip right off. Core the tomatoes and gently squeeze out the seeds. Chop half of them coarsely and in a food processor puree the other half.

2. In a large mixing bowl, combine the puree and chopped tomatoes. Blend the remaining ingredients, except the herb croutons, with the tomatoes. Cover and refrigerate for several hours. Serve chilled; garnish with herb croutons.

Serves 6.
Nutritional analysis, per serving: calories, 148; fat, 5g; carbohydrate, 14g; protein, 2g; calories from fat, 30%

Used with permission from the Florida Tomato Committee.

Gingered Carrot Soup

• •

2 pounds carrots

4 cups water

1 tablespoon butter or oil

1½ cups chopped onion

2 medium cloves garlic, minced

2 tablespoons freshly grated ginger

1½ teaspoons salt

¼ teaspoon cumin

¼ teaspoon ground fennel

¼ teaspoon cinnamon

¼ teaspoon allspice

¼ teaspoon dried mint

3 to 4 tablespoons fresh lemon juice

1 cup lightly toasted cashews

Buttermilk for garnish (optional)

1. Peel and trim carrots, and cut them into 1-inch chunks. Place in a medium-large saucepan with water; cover and bring to a boil. Lower the heat and simmer until very tender, about 10 to 15 minutes, depending on the size of the carrot pieces.
2. Meanwhile, heat the butter or oil in a small skillet. Add onions, and cook over medium heat for about 5 minutes. Add garlic, ginger, salt, and spices. Turn heat to low and continue to cook for another 8 to 10 minutes, or until everything is well mingled and the onions are very soft. Stir in lemon juice.
3. Use a food processor or blender to puree everything together (including the toasted cashews). You will need to do this in several batches. Transfer the puree to a kettle, and heat gently just before serving. If desired, pass a small pitcher of buttermilk for individual drizzling.

Serves 6 to 8.
Nutritional analysis, per serving: calories, 240; fat, 13g; cholesterol, 0mg; carbohydrate, 28g; fiber, 6g; protein, 6g; calories from fat, 20%

Gypsy Soup

• •

2 medium-size ripe tomatoes	2 teaspoons mild paprika
2 tablespoons olive oil	1 teaspoon turmeric
2 cups chopped onion	1 teaspoon basil
3 medium-size cloves garlic, crushed	Dash of cinnamon
	Dash of cayenne
1 stalk celery, minced	1 bay leaf
2 cups sweet potato, peeled and diced	3 cups water
	1 medium-size bell pepper, diced
1 teaspoon salt	1½ cups cooked chickpeas

1. In a medium saucepan, heat water to boiling. Core the tomatoes and plunge them into boiling water for a slow count of 10. Remove the tomatoes and peel them over the sink. Cut them open; squeeze out and discard the seeds. Chop the remaining pulp and set aside.

2. In a skillet or Dutch oven, heat olive oil over medium heat. Add onion, garlic, celery, and sweet potato, and cook over medium heat for about 5 minutes. Add salt and cook 5 minutes more. Add seasonings and water, cover, and simmer about 15 minutes.

3. Add tomato pulp, bell pepper, and chickpeas. Cover and simmer for about 10 more minutes, or until the vegetables are as tender as you like them. Taste to adjust the seasonings and serve.

Serves 4 to 5.

Nutritional analysis, per serving: calories, 290; fat, 9g; cholesterol, 0mg; carbohydrate, 47g; fiber, 10g; protein, 9g; calories from fat, 14%

Maine Wild Blueberry Soup

· ·

4½ cups fresh wild blueberries   ¼ cup honey
1 cup Pinot Noir   Vanilla crème fraîche for garnish

In a food processor, combine the blueberries, Pinot Noir, and honey; blend until the mixture becomes smooth, do not strain. Chill the soup before serving. Garnish each soup bowl with Vanilla crème fraîche.

Serves 4.
Nutritional analysis, per serving: calories, 234; fat, 5g; cholesterol, 0mg; fiber, 4g; protein, 2g; calories from fat, 19%

Used with permission from Chef William W. Sellner Jr., Ivy Manor Inn, Michelle's Fine Dining, Bar Harbor, Maine.

Shiitake Mushroom Miso Soup

· ·

½ cup Chinese cabbage (bok choy),   2 tablespoons miso paste (dark red)
  shredded   ½ cup tofu
1 ounce shiitake mushrooms   2½ tablespoons wakame seaweed
1 teaspoon sesame oil   flakes
6 cups water   ¼ cup scallion, bulbs and greens,
2½ tablespoons miso paste (Mello   thinly sliced
  White)

In a large pot, cook the bok choy and mushrooms in sesame oil. Add water, Mello White and dark red miso, tofu, and seaweed. Bring to a boil and simmer for 10 minutes. Rest soup for 5 minutes and serve with scallions.

Serves 4.
Nutritional analysis, per serving: calories, 83; fat, 4g; cholesterol, 0mg; carbohydrate, 7g; fiber, 1g; protein, 4g; calories from fat, 4%

Courtesy of Daniel Nadeau, M.D.

Vegetable Broth

1 tablespoon butter or
   margarine
½ cup chopped onion
½ cup diced turnip
½ cup diced parsley
1 cup diced celery, plus some inner
   leaves
1 bay leaf
½ teaspoon thyme
½ teaspoon salt, if desired

1 cup shredded salad greens
   (optional)
Vegetable scraps such as tomato
   skins, potato peelings, and
   mushroom bits
3 sprigs of parsley
2 whole cloves garlic
Dash of cayenne or to taste
Water and/or vegetable cooking
   liquid to cover

1. In a large, heavy saucepan, melt the butter or margarine over medium heat. Add the onion and cook for 3 to 5 minutes, until they brown.
2. Add the remaining ingredients to the pan, bring the broth to a boil, reduce the heat, and simmer the broth with the pan partially covered for 30 minutes to 1½ hours (the longer the better).
3. Strain the broth through a fine sieve, pressing the solids to extract the liquid.

Makes 4 to 6 cups.
Nutritional analysis, per serving: calories, 79; fat, 2g; carbohydrate, 14g; calories from fat, 23%

SALADS

Five-Fruit Salad

....

1 cup seedless grapes
½ cup orange, peeled, sliced, and
   quartered
½ cup cantaloupe, cubed
½ cup banana, sliced

½ cup pineapple chunks
¼ cup orange juice concentrate
1 teaspoon lime juice
2 teaspoons mint leaves, chopped
¼ teaspoon lime peel, grated

In a medium-size bowl, combine all ingredients; mix well.

Serves 4.
Nutritional analysis, per serving: calories, 101; fat, 1g; cholesterol, 0mg;
carbohydrate, 25g; fiber, 2g; protein, 1g; calories from fat, 3%

Used with permission from the California Table Grape Commission.

Practically Perfect Picnic Salad

....

1 cup seedless grapes
1 can (15 ounces) white beans,
   drained
½ cup celery, diced
¼ cup green onions, minced

2 tablespoons parsley, chopped
¼ cup lemon mustard dressing
   (recipe below)
1 package (10 ounces) lettuce
   leaves

1. In a large bowl, combine all ingredients except lettuce and dressing;
   mix well.
2. To serve, line plates with lettuce leaves and scoop salad onto each
   plate; drizzle with lemon mustard dressing.

Lemon Mustard Dressing: In a medium-size bowl, combine 2 tablespoons vegetable oil, 2 tablespoons lemon juice, 1 tablespoon Dijon mustard, ¼ teaspoon salt, and ¼ teaspoon pepper. Makes ¼ cup.

Serves 4.
Nutritional analysis, per serving: calories, 248; fat, 8g; cholesterol, 0mg; carbohydrate, 37g; fiber, 9g; protein, 10g; calories from fat, 22%

Used with permission from the California Table Grape Commission.

Coolin' Countrywild Rice Salad

1 cup rice, cooked according to package directions

1 red bell pepper, seeded and diced

1 green bell pepper, seeded and diced

1 can (2.25 ounces) sliced black olives, drained (¼ cup)

1 stalk celery, finely chopped (1¼ cup)

4 green onions, finely chopped (1¼ cup)

2 cans (6 ounces) crabmeat, drained and flaked (1 cup)

2 tablespoons lemon juice

1 teaspoon curry powder

½ cup nonfat or low-fat mayonnaise

In a large bowl, combine cooked, cooled rice and all ingredients; toss lightly. Chill and serve on a bed of lettuce and garnish with bell pepper sliver and olives.

Makes 6 cups.
Nutritional analysis, per serving: calories, 230; fat, 7g; cholesterol, 40mg; carbohydrate, 31g; fiber, 4g; protein, 14g; calories from fat, 10%

Used with permission from Lundberg Family Farms.

Southwestern Rice Salad

1 cup rice, cooked according to package directions

1 can (8.25 ounces) corn, drained (or 1 cup fresh or frozen)

1 can (15 ounces) black beans, rinsed (1¼ cup)

1 can (12 ounces) mild salsa (1¼ cup)

1 large tomato, seeded and diced (1 cup)

1 bunch green onions, diced (¾ cup)

1 green bell pepper, seeded and diced

1 red bell pepper, seeded and diced

1 can (2.25 ounces) sliced black olives, drained (¼ cup)

2 teaspoons cumin powder

¼ cup fresh cilantro, chopped (optional)

2 cloves garlic, minced

2 tablespoons lime juice

In a large bowl, combine cooked, cooled rice with all the ingredients; toss lightly. Chill and serve.

Makes 8 cups.
Nutritional analysis, per serving: calories, 180; fat, 2g; cholesterol, 0mg; fiber, 5g; protein, 6g; calories from fat, 2%

Used with permission from Lundberg Family Farms.

Anne's West 57th Street Salad

2 cups packed romaine lettuce, torn into pieces

2 cups packed spinach leaf, torn into pieces

2 Roma tomatoes, cut into bite size pieces, seeds removed

6 Calamata olives, pitted

¼ cup dried English walnuts, broken into small pieces

2 extra-large hard boiled eggs, sliced

½ cup croutons or rye bread cubes

2 cups light tuna in water, drained

1 tablespoon balsamic vinegar

1 tablespoon olive oil

In a large bowl, combine all ingredients; toss well.

Serves 4.
Nutritional analysis, per serving: calories, 250; fat, 13g; cholesterol, 145mg; carbohydrate, 8g; fiber, 2g; protein, 26g; calories from fat, 20%

Courtesy of Mary Fleming.

Artichoke and Roasted Red Pepper Salad with Roasted Red Pepper Dressing

Salad:

8 medium artichokes, cooked

4 red bell peppers

Lettuce leaves

½ cup sliced red onion

½ cup sliced ripe olives

Dressing:

1 roasted red bell pepper, reserved
from salad preparation

⅓ cup balsamic vinegar

¼ cup white wine or cider vinegar

2 cloves garlic, minced

1 tablespoon chopped fresh basil or
1 teaspoon dried basil

1 teaspoon chopped fresh rosemary
or ½ teaspoon dried rosemary

1 teaspoon sugar

1. Halve artichokes lengthwise; scoop out center petals and fuzzy centers. Remove outer leaves and reserve to garnish salad, or to use for snacks another time. Trim out hearts and slice thinly. Cover and set aside.
2. Place whole bell peppers under preheated broiler; broil under high heat until charred on all sides, turning frequently with tongs. Remove from oven; place in a paper bag for 15 minutes to steam skins. Trim off stems of peppers; remove seeds and ribs. Strip off skins; slice peppers into julienne strips. Reserve ¼ of the bell pepper strips to prepare dressing.
3. To assemble the salads: Arrange lettuce on 8 salad plates. Arrange sliced artichoke hearts, remaining bell pepper strips, red onion, and olive slices on lettuce. Garnish with a couple of cooked artichoke leaves, if desired.
4. For the dressing: In a blender or food processor container, combine the reserved bell pepper strips, vinegars, garlic, basil, rosemary, and sugar. Cover and process until well blended and nearly smooth. Spoon dressing over salads.

Serving suggestion: Assemble salads up to 4 hours ahead; chill dressing and spoon over salads just before serving.

Serves 8.
Nutritional analysis, per serving: calories, 88; fat, 1g; carbohydrate, 19g; cholesterol, 0mg; fiber, 5g; calories from fat, 12%

Courtesy of the California Artichoke Advisory Board.

Creamy Carrot Salad

• •

1 pound carrots, coarsely grated
2 medium-size apples, peeled and
   grated
1 cup firm yogurt*
1 tablespoon honey

A pinch of celery seed
Juice from 1 lemon
½ teaspoon salt
A few dashes ground pepper

Optional Variations (try using several together):

1 tablespoon toasted sesame seeds
¼ cup toasted sunflower seeds,
   almonds, or cashews

½ cup finely minced celery
½ cup chopped fresh pineapple
A handful of raisins

*If desired, substitute ½ cup yogurt
  and ½ cup mayonnaise.

1. In a large bowl, mix together the carrots and apples (and celery or
   pine nuts, if using these).
2. Blend together the yogurt and mayonnaise (if using), honey, celery
   seed, lemon juice, salt, and pepper, and add to the carrot-apple mixture. Add the optional seeds or nuts. Mix well and chill.

Serves 4 to 6.
Nutritional analysis, per serving (without optional ingredients): calories,
90; fat, 0g; cholesterol, 0mg; carbohydrate, 20g; fiber, 3g; protein, 3g;
calories from fat, 0%

Used with permission from Linda Welles, *The Genesis Farm Cookbook.*

Moroccan Quinoa Salad with Dressing

Salad:

4 cups boiling salted water

2 cups quinoa (wash well; quinoa has a natural coating that is very bitter)

3 tablespoons cumin powder

2 cloves garlic, minced

1 cup dried currants or raisins, soaked in warm water until soft

1 red onion, diced

4 stalks celery, diced

Dressing:

Juice of 3 lemons

½ teaspoon salt (sea salt preferred)

⅓ cup olive oil, extra-virgin preferred

1 tablespoon roasted cumin seeds

¼ cup roasted sunflower seeds for garnish

A thin slice of lemon for garnish

1. For the salad: In a large pot, add the quinoa, cumin, and garlic to the boiling water. Return to a boil, reduce the heat to a gentle simmer, cover, and cook until all the water is absorbed, about 20 minutes. Put the quinoa in a bowl and allow to cool.

2. Drain the softened currants and toss them into the cooked, cooled quinoa along with the onion and celery.

3. For the dressing: In a small bowl, combine the lemon juice and salt. Whisk rapidly while slowly pouring in the olive oil. Whisk until well mixed.

4. Toss the dressing with the salad and allow it to sit for at least 10 minutes. Toss the salad again before serving and garnish with roasted seeds and lemon slice.

Serves 6 to 10.
Nutritional analysis, per serving: calories, 350; fat, 15g; cholesterol, 0mg; carbohydrate, 50g; fiber, 5g; protein, 8g; calories from fat, 23%

Used with permission from Robin Byrne, *The Genesis Farm Cookbook.*

Orange and Fennel Salad

••

4 navel oranges

2 medium-size fennel bulbs

1 small red onion

4 tablespoons extra-virgin olive oil

Freshly ground pepper

1. Using a knife, peel the oranges and remove all of the white pith. With a sharp knife cut along the membranes separating the segments to remove them.
2. Wash the fennel and remove the green stalks and any bruised or discolored outer leaves. With a knife, slice the fennel crosswise as thinly as possible. Peel the onion and remove both ends. Slice the onion crosswise as thinly as possible.
3. In a medium-size bowl, combine the orange, fennel, and onion, and toss with olive oil. Serve the salad with freshly grated pepper, alone or over a bed of lettuce.

Serves 4 to 6.
Nutritional analysis, per serving: calories, 130; fat, 6g; cholesterol, 0mg; carbohydrate, 18g; fiber, 7g; protein, 5g; calories from fat, 9%

Used with permission from Sims Brannon.

Pomegranate Salad

· ·

3 cups spinach leaves, chopped

2 cups leafy green lettuce, torn

1 tablespoon olive oil

Ground pepper, to taste

¼ cup pomegranate seeds

2 tablespoons lemon juice

2 tablespoons toasted pine nuts

  (optional)

In a salad bowl, combine spinach and lettuce leaves. Drizzle with oil and season with pepper; toss to mix. Sprinkle with pomegranate seeds, lemon juice, and toasted pine nuts, if desired. (In a skillet, toast pine nuts over medium heat until golden brown, tossing constantly.)

Serves 4.
Nutritional analysis, per serving (without pine nuts): calories, 73; fat, 4g; cholesterol, 0mg; fiber, 0mg; calories from fat, 43%

Used with permission from the Produce for Better Health Foundation.

Raw Corn Salad Medley

4 ears fresh Supersweet corn
1 can (19 ounces) black beans, rinsed and drained
1 large tomato, chopped (about 1¼ cup)
3 tablespoons thinly sliced green onion (scallion)

2 tablespoons chopped fresh cilantro
3 tablespoons olive oil
2 tablespoons lime juice
½ teaspoon salt
½ teaspoon sugar

1. Cut kernels from cobs (makes about 2 cups). In a large bowl, combine kernels with beans, tomato, green onion, and cilantro.
2. In a small bowl, whisk together olive oil, lime juice, salt, and sugar until blended. Pour dressing over corn mixture; toss well to coat.

Serves 4.
Nutritional analysis, per serving: calories, 330; fat, 13g; cholesterol, 0mg; carbohydrate, 48g; fiber, 12g; protein, 12g; calories from fat, 20%

Used with permission from the Southern Supersweet Corn Council.

Red Cabbage Salad with Dressing

∙∙

Salad:

1 head red cabbage, thinly sliced

1 teaspoon salt (sea salt preferred)

1 red onion, thinly sliced

1 bunch parsley, minced

Dressing:

Juice from 2 lemons

¼ cup red wine vinegar

2 teaspoons prepared mustard

1 clove garlic, minced

¼ to ½ cup olive oil (extra-virgin preferred)

1. To make the salad: In a large bowl, combine the cabbage and salt; toss well and set aside to wilt for about 30 minutes.
2. Add the red onion and parsley.
3. To make the dressing: In a shallow bowl, combine the lemon juice, vinegar, mustard, and garlic.
4. Add the olive oil in a slow steady stream while rapidly stirring with a small whisk or fork.
5. Add the dressing to the salad and adjust the seasonings.

Serves 4 to 6.

Nutritional analysis, per serving: calories, 240; fat, 18g; cholesterol, 0mg; carbohydrate, 18g; fiber, 5g; protein, 4g; calories from fat, 28%

Used with permission from Robin Byrne, *The Genesis Farm Cookbook*.

Spinach Salad with Tarragon Vinegar and Toasted Almonds

∙∙∙

¾ cup dried almonds, slivered

1½ pounds spinach leaves, washed and torn into bite-size pieces

¼ cup tarragon vinegar

In a small skillet, toast the almonds over medium heat. Add the spinach and vinegar; toss well.

Serves 4.

Nutritional analysis, per serving: calories, 160; fat, 11g; cholesterol, 0mg; carbohydrate, 10g; fiber, 7g; protein, 9g; calories from fat, 17%

Used with permission from the Ellsworth Cooking School, Ellsworth, Maine.

Sweet Potato Black Bean Salad

∙∙∙

1 pound sweet potatoes, cubed and cooked

1½ cups black beans

1 cup roasted bell peppers (combine red, yellow, and green), julienned

1 medium-size ripe papaya, peeled and sliced

¾ cup watercress

½ cup chopped purple onion

½ teaspoon chili powder

3 tablespoons garlic-flavored oil

2 tablespoons red wine vinegar

¼ teaspoon hot pepper sauce

In a large bowl, combine all ingredients; toss to blend. Cover and let stand at room temperature for 25 minutes or refrigerate for 1 hour. To serve, spoon onto fresh greens and garnish with crisp fried tortilla strips.

Serves 8.

Nutritional analysis, per serving: calories, 173; fat, 5g; cholesterol, 0mg; carbohydrate, 27g; protein, 4g; calories from fat, 26%

Used with permission from the North Carolina SweetPotato Commission.

Tomato and Cannellini Salad

··

1 pound fresh tomatoes, cored and cut into chunks (makes about 3 cups)

1 can (19 ounces) cannellini beans (white kidney beans), rinsed and drained

¾ cup chopped onion

2 tablespoons chopped parsley

⅓ cup prepared Italian salad dressing

½ cup diced feta cheese (about 3 ounces)

In a medium-size bowl, combine tomatoes, cannellini beans, onion, parsley, and Italian dressing; toss until well coated. Cover; marinate for 15 minutes. Top with feta cheese. Serve over Romaine lettuce, if desired.

Serves 4.

Nutritional analysis, per serving: calories, 286; fat, 14g; carbohydrate, 29g; protein, 9g; calories from fat, 44%

Used with permission from the Florida Tomato Committee.

Watercress Salad with Pears, Celery, and Potatoes

Salad:

2 bunches watercress, washed, spun dry, and the stems removed

1 medium-size potato, peeled, cubed, and cooked until tender

1 stalk celery, thinly sliced on the diagonal

2 Bartlett pears, thinly sliced

½ cup chopped walnuts

Dressing:

¼ cup red wine vinegar

2 tablespoons balsamic vinegar

A pinch of salt and pepper

¼ teaspoon onion powder

¼ cup olive oil (extra-virgin preferred)

1. To make the salad: Form a bed of watercress on a serving platter.
2. Toss the potato and celery with half the vinaigrette.
3. Place the potato and celery on the bed of watercress, and top with pear slices and walnuts.
4. Drizzle the remaining dressing over the salad.
5. To make the dressing: Whisk all the ingredients together until they are well blended.

Serves 4.

Nutritional analysis, per serving: calories, 320; fat, 24g; cholesterol, 0mg; carbohydrate, 25g; fiber, 4g; protein, 4g; calories from fat, 36%

Used with permission from Robin Byrne, *The Genesis Farm Cookbook.*

ENTREES

California Avocado Tacos

1 medium-size onion, julienned

2 large green bell peppers, julienned

2 large red bell peppers, julienned

1 ripe avocado, peeled and seeded

12 flour tortillas

1½ cups fresh tomato salsa (see below)

1 cup fresh cilantro, finely chopped

Fresh tomato salsa:

1 cup tomatoes, diced

⅓ cup onions, diced

½ clove garlic, minced

2 teaspoons cilantro

⅓ teaspoon jalapeño peppers, chopped

½ teaspoon lime, juiced

Pinch of cumin

1. To make the tacos: Spray skillet with cooking spray and lightly cook onion and green and red peppers. Cut avocado into 12 slices. Warm tortillas in oven and fill with peppers, onions, avocado slices, salsa, and cilantro. Fold tortillas and serve.
2. To make the salsa: In a medium-size bowl, mix all the ingredients and refrigerate in advance.

Serves 12.
Nutritional analysis, per serving: calories, 170; fat, 6g; cholesterol, 3mg; calories from fat, 32%

Used with permission from the California Avocado Commission.

Chicken Breasts with California Avocado Risotto

••

Avocado Risotto:

1 tablespoon olive oil

2 cups fresh green bell pepper, diced

½ cup frozen corn

1½ cups fresh tomato, diced

4 cups white rice, cooked

¾ cup chopped fresh basil

½ medium avocado, diced

Chicken:

6 boneless, skinless chicken breasts (3 ounces each)

1 tablespoon olive oil

½ cup capers

¾ cup fresh lemon juice

½ cup chopped fresh parsley

½ medium-size avocado, sliced for garnish

1. To make the avocado risotto: In a skillet, heat olive oil over low heat and cook the green pepper, corn, and tomato for approximately 5 minutes.
2. Add the precooked white rice and basil. Simmer for approximately 5 more minutes and set aside. Add the diced avocado.
3. To make the chicken: Cook the chicken breasts in olive oil for approximately 5 minutes on each side over low heat.
4. Remove the chicken from the skillet and set aside. In the same skillet, cook the capers for approximately 1 minute. Remove from heat; add lemon juice and parsley.
5. To serve, place the risotto mixture on a plate and top with chicken breast. Pour the caper-and-lemon-juice mixture over the chicken and rice. Garnish with the avocado slices.

Serves 6.

Nutritional analysis, per serving: calories, 452; fat, 13g; cholesterol, 72mg; carbohydrate, 52g; fiber, 3g; protein, 32g; calories from fat, 26%

Used with permission from the California Avocado Commission.

Couscous with Chicken, Citrus, and Scallions

1 teaspoon olive or vegetable oil
½ pound chicken breast, sliced
4 scallions (green onions), diced
1 cup low-sodium chicken broth
½ cup canned mandarin oranges,
   drained and rinsed

½ grapefruit, peeled and sliced into
   small pieces, with pith removed
1 box (5.7 ounces) couscous, cooked
   (follow instructions on box)
1 tablespoon sliced almonds,
   toasted*

1. In a large pan, heat oil over medium-high heat and then add chicken slices. Brown them lightly on all sides, making sure they're cooked throughout. Remove and set aside.
2. Add scallions to pan and cook them for 5 to 10 minutes, until tender. Stir in broth and bring to a simmer. Stir in orange and grapefruit segments and chicken, and simmer for 5 minutes until all ingredients are heated throughout.
3. Add cooked couscous and stir well. Sprinkle with toasted almonds and serve.

*To toast almonds, spread them in a small pan and bake at 350°F for just 5 to 6 minutes, stirring once, until they have developed a pale brown color.

Serves 2.
Nutritional analysis, per serving: calories, 550; fat, 7g; cholesterol, 67mg; fiber, 6g; calories from fat, 12%

Used with permission from the Produce for Better Health Foundation.

Grilled Free-Range Chicken Breasts
•••

1 pound chicken breasts, boneless	¼ teaspoon salt
2 tablespoons olive oil	¼ teaspoon freshly ground pepper

1. Brush the chicken breasts with olive oil and sprinkle lightly with salt and pepper.
2. Meanwhile, preheat the grill. Before placing the chicken on the grill, coat it with cooking spray. Cook one side of the chicken for 5 minutes before turning it over. After you turn the chicken over, cook it another 5 minutes longer, until chicken is no longer pink on the inside. Remove from the grill and serve immediately.

Serves 4.
Nutritional analysis, per serving: calories, 250; fat, 17g; cholesterol, 75mg; carbohydrate, 0g; fiber, 0g; protein, 24g; calories from fat, 27%

To be served with Rosemary Roasted Sweet Potatoes (page 271) and Sesame Kale (page 269).

Courtesy of Daniel Nadeau, M.D.

Wild Blueberry Chicken Breasts

· ·

4 skinless, boneless chicken breast
  halves
½ teaspoon Cajun spices
2 teaspoons olive oil
3 cloves garlic, finely chopped
1 medium-size onion, finely
  chopped

⅓ cup red wine
2 cups fresh or frozen wild
  blueberries
1 teaspoon grated lemon rind
¼ teaspoon salt, optional

1. Dust chicken breasts with Cajun spices. In a skillet, heat olive oil over medium-high heat and cook chicken for 7 to 10 minutes, until brown and almost cooked through. (If the chicken breasts are thick, cover and cook 3 to 4 minutes longer.) Remove chicken breasts from pan and keep warm.

2. In the same pan, cook garlic and onion over medium heat for 3 to 5 minutes, until they become transparent, scraping the remaining bits of chicken from the bottom of the pan. Add red wine and cook down until most of the liquid evaporates. Add wild blueberries, lemon rind, and salt; simmer for 5 minutes. (If blueberries are frozen, cook until heated throughout.) Season with salt and pepper. Turn off the heat and let the mixture sit for 5 minutes to allow the flavors to blend. Spoon the mixture over the chicken breasts and serve immediately.

Serves 4.
Nutritional analysis, per serving: calories, 190; fat, 6g; cholesterol, 40mg; carbohydrate, 15g; fiber, 3g; protein, 16g; calories from fat, 10%

Used with permission from the Wild Blueberry Association of North America.

Baja Vegetable Stew

• •

2 hot red chili peppers, chopped and seeded

4 teaspoons olive oil

1 cup yellow onions, chopped

2 cloves garlic, minced

1 teaspoon ground cumin seed

3 medium-size tomatoes, halved, seeded, and chopped

2 cups low-sodium vegetable broth

1 red bell pepper, cut into 1-inch cubes

1 yellow bell pepper, cut into 1-inch cubes

2 zucchini, halved and diced

1 cup fresh, canned, or frozen corn

Salt and freshly ground pepper

2 cups black beans without salt

1 cup kidney beans

¾ teaspoon cider vinegar

1. In a skillet, roast chilies for 20 to 30 seconds over high heat. Remove from heat, cool, and remove seeds.
2. In a large pot, heat 2 teaspoons olive oil over medium-high heat. Add onions and cook 3 to 4 minutes, until a light golden brown. Add garlic and cumin, and cook, stirring, for 30 seconds. Add tomatoes, vegetable broth, and chilies, and simmer for 30 minutes, stirring occasionally. Remove from heat and let cool.
3. In a blender or food processor, puree the mixture until smooth. Pour mixture through a fine sieve or food mill. In a skillet, heat the remaining 2 teaspoons olive oil over medium-high heat. Add the bell peppers, zucchini, and corn. Season with salt and pepper and cook for 4 minutes. Add the black beans, kidney beans, and tomato mixture, and simmer for 1 to 2 minutes, until the vegetables are tender. Stir in the vinegar and garnish with cilantro, lime wedges, and avocado.

Serves 6.
Nutritional analysis, per serving: calories, 221; fat, 4g; cholesterol, 0mg; carbohydrate, 38g; fiber, 10g; protein, 11g; calories from fat, 7%

Used with permission from the Ellsworth Cooking School, Ellsworth, Maine.

Colorful Vegetable Fajitas

8 flour tortillas (8-inch diameter)

2 tablespoons vegetable oil

1 small red onion, peeled and cut into thin strips

1 small red bell pepper, seeded and sliced thin

1 small green bell pepper, seeded and sliced thin

1 teaspoon minced garlic

1 medium yellow summer squash, cut into 2-inch strips

½ cup salsa or picante sauce

1 teaspoon ground cumin

½ teaspoon salt

1 cup shredded Monterey Jack cheese

¼ cup chopped fresh cilantro

1. Wrap tortillas in aluminum foil and place in oven. Turn heat to 350°F. Bake for 15 minutes or until thoroughly heated.
2. In a 10-inch skillet, heat oil over medium-high heat. Add onions, red and green peppers, and garlic; stir to coat with oil. Cover, reduce heat to medium, and cook for 5 minutes. Stir squash into vegetables. Stir in salsa, cumin, and salt. Cover and cook for 5 minutes.
3. Spoon vegetable mixture evenly down the centers of warm tortillas and sprinkle with cheese and cilantro. Roll up tortillas and serve.

Serves 4.

Nutritional analysis, per serving: calories, 530; fat, 23g; cholesterol, 25mg; carbohydrate, 66g; fiber, 6g; protein, 17g; calories from fat, 35%

Submitted by Jessie, courtesy of Allrecipes.com.

Crunchy Vegetable Burrito Banditos

• •

½ cup shredded carrots
½ cup chopped broccoli
½ cup chopped cauliflower
2 green onions, thinly sliced
4 ounces shredded low-fat Cheddar
  cheese

¼ cup nonfat ranch-style salad
  dressing
½ teaspoon chili powder
4 flour tortillas (7-inch diameter)
1 cup green leaf lettuce, torn into
  bite-size pieces

1. In a mixing bowl, combine carrots, broccoli, cauliflower, and onions with cheese, ranch dressing, and chili powder.
2. On the counter, lay the tortillas flat and spoon about ½ cup vegetable mixture and ¼ cup lettuce down the center. Wrap each tortilla around the vegetable mixture.

Serves 4.
Nutritional analysis, per serving: calories, 204; fat, 7g; cholesterol, 20mg; carbohydrate, 22g; protein, 10g; calories from fat, 31%

Used with permission from Dole Food Company, Inc.

Sweet Pepper Vegetarian Chili

4 tablespoons olive oil

1 medium-size onion, diced

1 medium-size carrot, diced

2 medium-size yellow bell peppers, diced

2 medium-size red bell peppers, diced

2 medium-size yellow squash, diced

2 medium-size zucchini, diced

1 can (28 ounces) chopped tomatoes

1 can (14.5 ounces) fat-free vegetable broth

1 can (15.5 ounces) black beans

1 can (15.5 ounces) red kidney beans

1 can (15.5 ounces) white beans (your choice)

4 tablespoons chili powder

1 tablespoon cumin

2 tablespoons fresh chopped cilantro

½ teaspoon cayenne pepper, optional

1. In a large stockpot, heat the olive oil over medium-high heat and cook the onion, carrot, and peppers until browned, about 8 minutes, stirring occasionally.
2. Add the squash and zucchini and cook through, another 6 to 8 minutes.
3. Add the tomatoes (including the liquid) and vegetable stock. Bring to a boil.
4. Drain the beans and add to the pot. Reduce heat and simmer for 15 minutes.
5. Add the chili powder, cumin, and cilantro.
6. Continue to simmer until the chili thickens, about 8 minutes.
7. Salt and pepper to taste. To add a little spice, add ½ teaspoon of cayenne pepper. Serve over brown or white rice, or enjoy with a dollop of fat-free sour cream.

Serves 6 to 8.
Nutritional analysis, per serving: calories, 370; fat, 12g; cholesterol, 0mg; carbohydrate, 52g; fiber, 17g; protein, 16g; calories from fat, 18%

Courtesy of Erik Zwillinger, Fedora Café, Lawrenceville, New Jersey.

California Rolls

• •

3 to 5 ounces nori seaweed, cut
lengthwise
6 tablespoons water
2 teaspoons white rice vinegar
10 ounces Sushi Rice (page 265)

2 teaspoons wasabi root or store-
bought wasabi paste
¼ cucumber, peeled, seeded, and
julienned
¼ avocado, thinly sliced
4 ounces blue crabmeat

1. In a large skillet, toast the nori, shiny side down, over high heat for 3 to 5 minutes.
2. To make the California roll: Put a bamboo mat in front of you so that it can easily be rolled away from you. Put the nori on the rolling mat shiny side down, with the long side running from left to right.
3. In a small bowl, combine the water and vinegar. Dip your hands in the bowl and scoop out a large ball of rice (about ¾ cup). Cover the entire surface of the nori with the rice as neatly as possible, since it will become the outside of the roll. Take the rice-covered nori and turn it over onto a wet towel. The rice will now be on the towel and the nori facing you. Run a streak of the wasabi paste from left to right down the middle of the nori. Lay the slices of cucumber, avocado, and crabmeat over the wasabi streak.
4. Grasp the towel in both hands, thumbs underneath, pressing lightly on the fillings with the index fingers of both hands. Lift the towel so that the edge of the nori closest to you meets the opposite end of the roll. Pick up the towel from the top of the roll. Slowly nudge the roll away from you, until no more nori is visible.
5. Cover the roll with the wet towel and place the bamboo mat over the towel. Apply pressure to the mat to square the roll off. Remove the mat and the wet cloth. Place the California roll on a cutting board, seam side down. Dip the tip of the knife in the bowl of water and vinegar; then slice the roll in half, using a swift back and forth cut. Clean the knife with a towel, dip the tip back in the water and vinegar and cut each half into thirds.

Serves 2.

Nutritional analysis, per serving: calories, 210; fat, 5g; cholesterol, 60mg; carbohydrate, 24g; fiber, 3g; protein, 17g; calories from fat, 8%

Courtesy of Daniel Nadeau, M.D.

Curried Eggplant with Spinach

4 tablespoons olive oil

1 tablespoon brown mustard

2 tablespoons dried sesame seeds

1 cup onion, chopped

12 cloves garlic, minced

1 pound spinach, chopped

2 eggplants, cut into ½-inch cubes

1 ginger root, peeled and grated

2 teaspoons ground turmeric

½ teaspoon paprika

2 teaspoons ground cumin

3 medium-size tomatoes, finely chopped

Salt and freshly ground pepper

4 tablespoons cilantro for garnish

1. In a large, deep skillet or Dutch oven, heat the olive oil, mustard, and sesame seeds over medium-high heat until the seeds begin to pop. Add the onions and garlic and cook until tender. Add the spinach, a small amount at a time, stirring constantly, to keep the spinach from scorching.
2. Once the spinach wilts, add the eggplant, ginger, turmeric, paprika, and cumin; cook until all the ingredients are blended. Cover and cook over medium-low heat for 15 minutes. Add the tomatoes and season with salt and pepper. Cook uncovered for 5 minutes longer. Garnish with cilantro and serve over rice.

Serves 4.

Nutritional analysis, per serving: calories, 290; fat, 18g; cholesterol, 0mg; carbohydrate, 31g; fiber, 12g; protein, 9g; calories from fat, 27%

Used with permission from the Ellsworth Cooking School, Ellsworth, Maine.

Haddock with Garlic and Olive Oil

••

2 tablespoons olive oil

6 cloves garlic, chopped

6 fresh or frozen haddock fillets, 4
ounces each

Fresh parsley for garnish

Spray a skillet with olive oil cooking spray and heat over medium heat. Add olive oil and garlic and cook for 3 to 5 minutes, until the garlic is soft. Add haddock and cook for 3 to 4 minutes on each side. Remove from pan and serve immediately. Garnish with fresh parsley.

Serves 6.
Nutritional analysis, per serving: calories, 140; fat, 5g; cholesterol, 65mg; carbohydrate, 1g; fiber, 0g; protein, 22g; calories from fat, 8%

Used with permission from the Ellsworth Cooking School, Ellsworth, Maine

Jim's Salmon Sergio

· ·

4 salmon steaks, 4 ounces each

2 tablespoons fresh lemon juice

2 potatoes (red or new), sliced

1 pound Roma tomatoes, diced

2 red bell peppers, diced

1 cup scallions, with bulbs and
greens, diced

4 cloves garlic, minced

2 tablespoons extra-virgin olive oil

1. In a large bowl, soak the salmon steaks with lemon juice and water for about 10 minutes. Rinse the fish, pat dry, and coat with a light dusting of flour.
2. In a separate bowl, combine the potatoes, tomatoes, red peppers, scallions, garlic, and olive oil. Set aside.
3. In a large skillet, combine the fish and vegetable mixture and cook over medium heat for 20 to 30 minutes. If you prefer, you can cook the vegetable mixture over medium heat for 10 minutes and then add the salmon steaks.

Serves 4.

Nutritional analysis, per serving: calories, 310; fat, 15g; cholesterol, 60mg; carbohydrate, 19g; fiber, 3g; protein, 25g; calories from fat, 23%

Courtesy of James A. Joseph, Ph.D.

Pan-Grilled Mushroom Fajitas

• •

½ teaspoon salt
1 pound fresh white mushrooms, cut in ¼-inch thick slices
8 ounces portobello caps, halved and cut in ¼-inch slices
1 teaspoon finely chopped garlic
2 tablespoons vegetable oil
1 large onion, cut in 8 wedges
1 large red bell pepper, cut in ½-inch strips
2 teaspoons finely chopped fresh jalapeño peppers
1 tablespoon chopped cilantro (optional)
8 low-fat tortillas (6-inch size), warmed

1. In a large skillet, sprinkle salt and heat over high heat until hot, about 5 minutes. Add mushrooms and garlic. Cook and stir until mushrooms are tender, about 3 minutes; remove to bowl.
2. In the same pan, add vegetable oil, onion, and red pepper. Cook and stir until tender, about 5 minutes. Return mushrooms to skillet; stir in jalapeño peppers and, if desired, 1 tablespoon chopped cilantro; heat until hot. Spoon an equal amount into the center of each tortilla; fold bottom and sides over filling. Serve with sour cream, salsa, lime wedges, and additional finely chopped jalapeño, if desired.

Serves 4.
Nutritional analysis, per serving: calories, 293; fat, 9g; carbohydrate, 49g; protein, 11g; calories from fat, 28%

Used with permission from the Mushroom Council.

Pasta e Fagioli with Basil

1 medium-size onion, chopped
4 cloves garlic, minced
½ pound mushrooms, sliced
1 red or gold sweet bell pepper, chopped
2 stalks celery, sliced
2 cans (14½ ounces) low-sodium, ready-cut tomatoes with juice
2 cans (15 ounces) cannellini beans, rinsed and drained

½ pound or ½ bunch chard or spinach, cleaned, stems removed, and leaves coarsely chopped
⅔ cup fresh basil
Salt and pepper to taste
1 pound ziti or other small chunky pasta, cooked al dente
Grated Parmesan for garnish

1. Coat a nonstick skillet with olive oil cooking spray. Cook onion, garlic, mushrooms, bell pepper, and celery over medium heat for 5 minutes or until soft.
2. Reduce heat and add tomatoes with juice and cannellini beans. Add water, if necessary, to desired consistency. Cover and simmer for 15 minutes. Add chard or spinach, basil, salt and pepper. Simmer 15 minutes longer. Toss with additional chopped basil to taste and serve over pasta. Sprinkle with grated Parmesan.

Serves 8.
Nutritional analysis, per serving: calories, 384; fat, 2g; cholesterol, 0mg; fiber, 9g; calories from fat, 5%

Used with permission from The Green House Fine Herbs.

Risotto by the Sea

6 cups chicken or vegetable stock

2 tablespoons butter or margarine

2 cloves garlic, minced, or ½
teaspoon garlic powder

1 pound large raw shrimp, shelled,
deveined, and cleaned

¼ teaspoon dried dill

Dash cayenne pepper

Dash ground nutmeg

2 tablespoons olive oil

1 large onion, chopped fine

2 cups white arborio rice

1 cup dry-fruity wine such as
Zinfandel or Chardonnay

¼ cup fresh parsley, washed and
chopped fine

1. In a stockpot, simmer 6 cups of stock.
2. Meanwhile, heat butter in a large skillet. When it begins to sizzle, add garlic and stir. Add raw shrimp and cook briefly (1 to 2 minutes on each side), until shrimp turn pink. Add dill, cayenne, and nutmeg. Add shrimp and juices to stock pot, and stir gently. Set aside shrimp and pan juices.
3. Heat olive oil in a thick-walled large pot over medium heat. Add onion and stir until translucent. Add rice and stir until rice is coated with oil. Add wine, ½ cup at a time, and stir until wine is nearly absorbed. Begin adding liquid ½ cup at a time, stirring after each addition. This takes approximately 15 minutes. Add liquid from shrimp, continue cooking and stir for another 5 minutes, or until rice is al dente and liquid is creamy. Stir shrimp and parsley into rice mixture. Top with Parmesan cheese, if desired.

Serves 4.

Nutritional analysis, per serving: calories, 440; fat, 11g; cholesterol, 115mg; carbohydrate, 56g; fiber, 1g; protein, 21g; calories from fat, 16%

Used with permission from Lundberg Family Farms.

Subji Biriyani (Vegetable-Rice Casserole)

1 cup basmati rice
½ cup moong dal*
5 cups water
¼ teaspoon turmeric
1½ teaspoons salt
¼ cup unsalted dry roasted peanuts
1 small onion
½ teaspoon cumin seeds
1 teaspoon cayenne pepper, optional
2 tablespoons oil

1 small potato, peeled and chopped into ¼-inch cubes
1 medium-size carrot, peeled and chopped into ¼-inch cubes
1 small tomato, chopped into ½-inch cubes
½ cup frozen peas
¼ cup cashews, chopped
¼ cup golden raisins
½ cup nonfat plain yogurt

1. Clean rice and moong dal of any extraneous material. Combine them and wash in 2 to 3 changes of water, until water is relatively clear. Strain and set aside.
2. In a 2 to 3 quart saucepan, add the rice and dal mixture, 3 cups of water, turmeric, and 1 teaspoon salt. Bring to a boil. Reduce heat to a simmer. Cover with lid, leaving a small crack open for steam to escape. Simmer for 12 to 15 minutes until all the water is absorbed and the rice is done.
3. Meanwhile, in a blender, coarsely grind peanuts and set aside.
4. To make the onion masala: In the same blender jar finely grind onions, cumin seeds, and cayenne pepper. (You may need to add 1 to 2 tablespoons water to be able to grind.) Set aside.
5. Heat a heavy nonstick 4-quart skillet and add ground onions. Cook for a few minutes until most of the water is evaporated. Add oil and fry until onion masala is light brown.
6. Add ground peanuts, chopped potatoes, carrots, tomatoes, peas, cashews, raisins, and ½ teaspoon salt. Mix well. Add 1 cup water, bring to a boil and reduce heat. Cover with a lid and simmer until vegetables are tender, about 8 to 10 minutes, stirring occasionally.
7. Whip yogurt lightly and add 1 tablespoon at a time to the vegetables, stirring constantly. Cook for 5 to 7 minutes without covering, stirring occasionally to blend the yogurt with the vegetables.
8. Add the remaining 1 cup water and bring to a boil.

9. Add the cooked rice and dal. Stir gently with spatula to avoid breaking rice. Cover with a lid and steam through for 2 to 3 minutes.

10. Remove from the heat, close the lid and let stand until ready to serve. Fluff with a fork before serving.

Serves 6.
Nutritional analysis, per serving: calories, 310; fat, 10g; cholesterol, 0mg; carbohydrate, 45g; fiber, 3g; protein, 9g; calories from fat, 29%

*Moong dal, a type of lentil, is available in health food stores and those specializing in Indian food.
"Subji Biriyani," from *New Indian Home Cooking* by Madhu Gadia, copyright © 1997 by Madhu Gadia; previously published as *Lite and Luscious Cuisine of India*. Used with permission of Berkley Publishing Group, a division of Penguin Putnam, Inc.

Sushi Rice

. . . .

2 cups short grain white rice   ½ cup white rice vinegar
2⅓ cups water

1. To wash the rice: In a large bowl, soak the rice in water. Stir the rice around in the bowl with your hand. After the water becomes cloudy, strain the rice and water. Transfer the rice back into the bowl and add fresh water and repeat the process. Keep washing the rice until the water is no longer cloudy, approximately 5 minutes. Finally, leave the washed rice in the strainer and let stand for 30 to 60 minutes until the excess water drains from the rice.

2. To cook the rice on a gas range: In a medium pot, add the rice and water; cover tightly and cook on medium-high heat until the rice steams, approximately 10 minutes. Turn the heat to high and cook 2 minutes longer. You may notice a white foam around the lid and the lid jiggling up and down. Reduce the heat to medium and cook 5 minutes

longer, until the foam stops and you hear a crackling sound. Turn the heat off and let the rice stand for 15 minutes, covered, as the rice steams.

3. Place the rice in a non-metal shallow pan. Sprinkle the vinegar over the steaming rice, tossing well. Cover the pan with a damp cloth. Let stand another 15 minutes, to cool.

4. To cook the rice on an electric range: Follow the above directions; however, to change the heating temperature, switch burners rather than adjusting the heat on the same burner.

5. To cook the rice in an electric rice cooker: Follow the instructions that came with the rice cooker.

Variation: If you are changing the amount of rice being cooked, it's very important that you change the size of the saucepan (one cup of rice should be cooked in a very small pan). Also, if you are not using a heavy saucepan, reduce the cooking time by watching for the signs of rice steaming, boiling (lid jiggling), and drying (crackling sound).

Serves 5.
Nutritional analysis, per serving: calories, 100; fat, 0g; cholesterol, 0mg; carbohydrate, 21g; fiber, 1g; protein, 2g; calories from fat, 0%

Courtesy of Daniel Nadeau, M.D.

Tomato Ratatouille Sauté

3 large, fresh tomatoes (about 1½ pounds)
1 tablespoon olive oil
1 cup onion, chopped
1½ teaspoons garlic, minced
2 cups zucchini, sliced
2 cups eggplant, diced

2 cups green bell pepper chunks
¼ teaspoon salt
1 teaspoon basil leaves, crushed
¼ teaspoon thyme leaves, crushed
¼ teaspoon ground black pepper
3 cups cooked long-grain rice

1. Use tomatoes held at room temperature until fully ripe. Core tomatoes, and chop coarsely (makes about 4 cups). Set aside. In a large saucepan, heat olive oil over medium-high heat until hot. Add onion and garlic; cook and stir until softened, about 3 to 4 minutes.
2. Add zucchini, eggplant, and green pepper; cook, stirring, until slightly softened, about 2 to 3 minutes. Add ½ cup water, salt, basil, thyme, black pepper, and tomatoes; bring to a boil; reduce heat and simmer, covered, until vegetables are tender, about 15 minutes, stirring occasionally. Serve over cooked rice.

Serves 4.
Nutritional analysis, per serving: calories, 316; fat, 5g; cholesterol, 0mg; fiber, 5g; calories from fat, 13%

Used with permission from the Florida Tomato Committee.

SIDE DISHES

Kale with Garlic
••

1 quart kale, chopped
8 cloves garlic, minced

2 teaspoons olive oil
Salt and freshly ground pepper

Spray the surface of a skillet with nonstick cooking spray and heat over medium-high. Add kale, garlic, and olive oil. Stirring frequently, cook for 4 to 5 minutes, until the kale wilts. Season with salt and pepper.

> **Serves 4.**
> Nutritional analysis, per serving: calories, 62; fat, 3g; cholesterol, 0mg; carbohydrate, 9g; fiber, 1g; protein, 3g; calories from fat, 4%

Courtesy of Daniel Nadeau, M.D.

Roasted Vegetables with Kale
••

2 large onions, cut into thick wedges
4 large potatoes, cut into 1-inch cubes
4 carrots, peeled and cut into 1-inch cubes
1 small butternut squash, peeled, seeded, and cut into 1-inch cubes
4 cups mixed vegetables such as

celeriac, parsnips, rutabagas, turnips, Jerusalem artichokes, and salsify, cubed
4 large cloves garlic, chopped fine and mashed into a paste with ½ teaspoon salt
¼ cup olive oil
Freshly ground pepper
8 cups washed and chopped kale

1. Preheat oven to 400°F.
2. In a large roasting pan, place the onions, potatoes, carrots, squash, and mixed root vegetables. In a small bowl, mix the garlic with the olive oil and pepper. With your hands, mix the garlic-oil combination

into the vegetables, coating them thoroughly. Roast the mixture for about 45 minutes, stirring occasionally, until the vegetables are tender.

3. Meanwhile, in a large soup pot, cook the kale over medium heat, using just enough water to keep it from burning, for about 10 minutes, stirring occasionally. The kale should be wilted and the water evaporated.

4. Mix the kale into the roasted vegetables and put on a serving platter.

Serves 6.

Nutritional analysis, per serving: calories, 340; fat, 10g; cholesterol, 0mg; carbohydrate, 59g; fiber, 10g; protein, 9g; calories from fat, 16%

Used with permission from Laura Greenspan, *The Genesis Farm Cookbook*.

Sesame Kale

· ·

4 cups kale, chopped   2 teaspoons olive oil
3 tablespoons dried sesame seeds   Salt and freshly ground pepper

Spray a nonstick skillet with cooking spray and heat the pan over medium-high. Add kale, sesame seeds, and olive oil to the pan. Cook for 4 to 5 minutes, stirring constantly, until the kale is wilted. Add salt and pepper to taste.

Serves 4.

Nutritional analysis, per serving: calories, 90; fat, 6g; cholesterol, 0mg; carbohydrate, 8g; fiber, 2g; protein, 3g; calories from fat, 9%

Used with permission from the Ellsworth Cooking School, Ellsworth, Maine.

Roasted Potatoes with Red Pepper and Onion

• •

5 small potatoes, each cut
    lengthwise into 6 wedges
1 tablespoon olive oil
Salt and freshly ground pepper

1 medium-size yellow onion, thinly
    sliced
1 red bell pepper, julienned

1. Pat dry the potatoes with paper towels and place them on a rectangular baking sheet with sides. Drizzle olive oil over the potatoes and sprinkle with salt and pepper; toss well. Bake at 450°F for 15 minutes. Remove potatoes from oven and toss well.
2. Place onions and peppers on top of the potatoes and bake 15 minutes longer, or until a fork inserted into the center of a potato wedge indicates they are done.

Serves 6.
Nutritional analysis, per serving: calories, 90; fat, 3g; cholesterol, 0mg; carbohydrate, 17g; fiber, 2g; protein, 2g; calories from fat, 4%

Used with permission from the Ellsworth Cooking School, Ellsworth, Maine.

Rosemary Roasted Sweet Potatoes

•••

2 pounds sweet potatoes, roughly
  cut into 1½-inch pieces
3 large cloves garlic, peeled and
  coarsely chopped
1 tablespoon chopped fresh
  rosemary

2 tablespoons olive oil
¼ cup toasted pine nuts
2 tablespoons chopped parsley
1 teaspoon salt
¼ teaspoon coarsely ground black
  pepper

In a roasting pan, combine sweet potatoes, garlic, rosemary, and olive oil; toss to blend well. Roast at 375°F for 40 minutes, turning sweet potatoes occasionally. Just before serving, season with pine nuts, parsley, salt, and pepper.

Serves 6.
Nutritional analysis, per serving: calories, 270; fat, 11g; cholesterol, 0mg; carbohydrate, 39g; fiber, 5g; protein, 4g; calories from fat, 17%

Used with permission from the North Carolina SweetPotato Commission.

Royal Basmati Rice

3 tablespoons olive oil

1 teaspoon whole cumin seeds (or ½ teaspoon powdered cumin)

1 large onion, peeled and chopped

2 cups brown basmati*

4 cups water or broth*

¼ teaspoon black pepper

½ teaspoon salt

½ cup frozen green peas

In a heavy skillet or Dutch oven with a lid, heat olive oil and cumin seeds over medium-high heat. Stir for a few seconds. Add onions and cook until translucent. Add rice and continue cooking for 3 to 4 minutes. Add liquid and bring to a boil. Cover and reduce heat to low and cook 45 to 50 minutes. Stir in peas the last few minutes of cooking.

*Substitution: white basmati can be substituted for brown by adjusting water to 3 cups.

Serves 4.
Nutritional analysis, per serving: calories, 310; fat, 10g; cholesterol, 0mg; carbohydrate, 53g; fiber, 4g; protein, 6g; calories from fat, 15%

Used with permission from Lundberg Family Farms.

Spanish Rice

• •

1 tablespoon olive oil
½ cup onions, chopped
1½ cups brown rice
1 small green bell pepper, diced
2 celery stalks, diced
4 ounces hot green chili peppers,
   diced

1 can (28 ounces) low-sodium,
   ready-cut tomatoes in juice
   (reserve juice and add enough
   water/broth to equal 3 cups
   liquid for later use)
2 cloves garlic, minced
⅛ teaspoon cayenne pepper

In a skillet or 3-quart saucepan, heat olive oil over medium-high heat. Add onion and garlic and cook for 3 to 5 minutes, until the onion is translucent. Add rice and cook for 1 minute. Add bell pepper, celery, chili peppers, tomatoes, and 3 cups liquid, including juice from tomatoes. Bring the mixture to a boil, reduce the heat and add cayenne pepper, and simmer for 50 minutes. The mixture should be creamy, not dry.

Serves 6.

Nutritional analysis, per serving: calories, 233; fat, 3g; cholesterol, 0mg; carbohydrate, 44g; fiber, 4g; protein, 6g; calories from fat, 11%

Used with permission from the Ellsworth Cooking School, Ellsworth, Maine.

Spinach Feta Rice

· ·

1 cup uncooked rice

1 cup vegetable or chicken broth

1 cup water

1 medium-size onion, chopped

1 cup (4 ounces) mushrooms, sliced

2 cloves garlic, minced

1 tablespoon lemon juice

½ teaspoon dried oregano leaves

6 cups spinach leaves, shredded

4 ounces feta cheese, crumbled

½ teaspoon freshly ground black pepper

¼ cup chopped pimiento (optional)

1. In a medium-size saucepan, bring rice, broth, and water to a boil. Stir, cover, reduce heat, and simmer for 15 to 20 minutes, or until rice is tender and liquid is absorbed.
2. In a large skillet coated with cooking spray, cook onion, mushrooms, and garlic over medium heat until onion is tender. Stir in lemon juice and oregano. Add to rice.
3. Add spinach, cheese, and pepper to rice; toss lightly until spinach is wilted. Garnish with chopped pimiento, if desired.

Serves 6.
Nutritional analysis, per serving: calories, 181; fat, 3g; cholesterol, 8mg; fiber, 3g; calories from fat, 14%

Used with permission from the Produce for Better Health Foundation.

Asparagus Brown Rice Oriental Medley

2 teaspoons canola oil

2 cups (12 ounce package) frozen
asparagus spears and tips,
thawed and drained

1 cup mushrooms, thinly sliced

½ cup onions, chopped

½ cup celery, thinly sliced

2 cups cooked brown rice

2 tablespoons light soy sauce

In a large nonstick fry pan or wok, heat the oil over medium-high heat. Add the asparagus, mushrooms, onions, and celery; cook, stirring, for 2 minutes. Add the brown rice and soy sauce; cook, stirring frequently, for 2 minutes longer. Remove from heat and serve immediately.

Serves 4.

Nutritional analysis, per serving: calories, 162; fat, 3g; cholesterol, 0mg; carbohydrate, 29g; fiber, 4g; calories from fat, 17%

Used with permission from the Michigan Asparagus Advisory Board.

Barley and Wheat-Berry Pilaf

· ·

1½ cups hulled barley, washed well

½ cup wheat berries, washed well

1 teaspoon cumin seeds

2 bay leaves

4 cloves garlic, minced

¼ teaspoon fresh grated ginger

Zest of ½ lemon

1 onion, diced

2 carrots, diced

2 stalks celery, diced

¼ cup raisins

½ cup fresh parsley, minced

A drizzle of olive oil

4 cups boiling vegetable stock

Salt to taste, if the stock is unsalted

1. Preheat the oven to 350°F.
2. Place all the ingredients in a 2-quart casserole, stir, cover, and bake for 40 to 60 minutes, until all the liquid is absorbed and barley is tender.

Serves 4 to 8.

Nutritional analysis, per serving: calories, 270; fat, 3g; cholesterol, 0mg; carbohydrate, 56g; fiber, 12g; protein, 9g; calories from fat, 4%

Used with permission from Robin Byrne, *The Genesis Farm Cookbook.*

Beautiful Beet Slaw

· ·

6 firm, fresh beets, scrubbed or
   peeled
4 carrots, scrubbed or peeled
1 cup sliced green cabbage
1 onion, thinly sliced into half
   moon shapes
1 bunch parsley, minced

3 tablespoons balsamic vinegar
2 tablespoons red wine vinegar
1 tablespoon grainy mustard
Salt and pepper to taste
⅓ cup olive oil, extra-virgin
   preferred

1. In a food processor or with a vegetable grater, grate the beets, carrots, cabbage, and onion. In a medium bowl, mix these together with the parsley and set aside.
2. In a small bowl, combine the vinegars, mustard, salt, and pepper and mix well with a whisk. As you continue to whisk, slowly pour in the olive oil until it is well emulsified.
3. Toss the dressing with the salad and adjust the seasoning if needed. Chill or serve at room temperature.

Serves 6 to 8.
Nutritional analysis, per serving: calories, 180; fat, 12g; cholesterol, 0mg; carbohydrate, 17g; fiber, 5g; protein, 3g; calories from fat, 19%

Used with permission from Robin Byrne, *The Genesis Farm Cookbook*.

Confetti Quinoa

••

1 cup raw quinoa

2 cups water

¼ teaspoon salt

½ medium-size onion, finely
chopped

¼ red bell pepper, seeded and
finely chopped

¼ green bell pepper, seeded and
finely chopped

1 teaspoon olive oil

2 tablespoons chopped or toasted
almonds or ¼ cup sliced water
chestnuts

2 tablespoons chopped fresh
coriander leaves

1. Rinse quinoa thoroughly in a fine sieve. Bring two cups of water to a boil, then add salt and quinoa and bring to a boil again. Cover, reduce heat to a low simmer, and cook for 15 minutes.

2. Meanwhile, in a skillet, cook onion and peppers in olive oil. Combine with grain. Just before serving, stir in almonds or water chestnuts and coriander leaves. Check salt.

Makes 3 cups.

Nutritional analysis, per serving: calories, 140; fat, 4g; cholesterol, 0mg; carbohydrate, 22g; fiber, 3g; protein, 4g; calories from fat, 6%

Grape and Wild Rice Stuffing

• •

1 can (14.5 ounces) vegetable broth	½ cup apple, chopped
½ cup water	1 tablespoon butter or margarine
½ cup brown rice	1 teaspoon fresh sage, minced
½ cup wild rice	¼ teaspoon pepper
½ cup onion, chopped	2 cups red seedless grapes
½ cup celery, chopped	Salt, to taste

1. In a large pot, bring broth and water to a boil. Add brown and wild rice. Bring to boil again, reduce heat, cover, and simmer for 45 to 55 minutes, until the rice is tender and the liquid is absorbed.
2. Meanwhile, in a skillet, cook the onion, celery, and apple in butter; add the sage and pepper. After the mixture is cooked, add the rice and grapes; mix well. Season with salt, if necessary.
3. Place the stuffing in a 1½ quart baking dish and bake at 350°F for 20 minutes or until heated throughout.

Serves 4 to 6.
Nutritional analysis, per serving: calories, 188; fat, 4g; cholesterol, 1mg; carbohydrate, 34g; fiber, 3g; protein, 7g; calories from fat, 15%

Used with permission from the California Table Grape Commission.

Red and Green Beans with Pine Nuts

1¼ pounds green snap beans, ends trimmed

2 teaspoons olive oil

¼ cup red onion, sliced

8 cloves garlic, peeled and chopped

1 red bell pepper, roasted, peeled, and sliced into 1-inch strips

6 ounces pine nuts, lightly toasted

¼ teaspoon salt

Dash black pepper

1. Wash beans and place in steamer kettle; cover and steam for 20 minutes. Taste the beans to see whether or not they are tender enough. If not, continue cooking for 5 to 10 minutes.
2. Meanwhile, spray a skillet with cooking spray. Heat olive oil over medium heat and cook onions and garlic until soft. Add prepared red pepper and cooked beans. Sprinkle with pine nuts, salt, and pepper. Toss to mix all the ingredients and transfer to a bowl. Serve warm.

Serves 6.
Nutritional analysis, per serving: calories, 260; fat, 20g; cholesterol, 0mg; carbohydrate, 13g; fiber, 6g; protein, 7g; calories from fat, 30%

Used with permission from the Ellsworth Cooking School, Ellsworth, Maine.

Skillet Corn Bread

• •

1 cup yellow cornmeal
¾ cup stone ground whole wheat
  flour
½ cup unbleached white flour
2 teaspoons baking powder
½ teaspoon baking soda

½ teaspoon salt
1 cup buttermilk, cultured from
  skim milk
¼ cup egg substitute
½ cup sugar
2 tablespoons canola oil

1. Preheat oven to 350°F. Spray a 9- or 10-inch cast-iron skillet with cooking spray.
2. In a medium-size bowl, combine the cornmeal, whole wheat flour, white flour, baking powder, baking soda, and salt.
3. In another medium-size bowl, combine buttermilk, egg substitute, sugar, and oil. Combine the ingredients from both bowls and mix thoroughly.
4. Spread the mixture in the pan and bake for 20 minutes, or until the center is firm to the touch. Serve hot, warm, or at room temperature.

Serves 9.
Nutritional analysis per serving: calories, 210; fat, 4g; cholesterol, 0mg; carbohydrate, 37g; fiber, 2g; protein, 5g; calories from fat, 7%

Used with permission from the Ellsworth Cooking School, Ellsworth, Maine.

Spring Greens and Polenta Pie

• •

2 tablespoons olive oil

½ cup chopped leeks, scallions, or
spring onions

2 cloves garlic, minced

12 cups chopped mixed spring
greens such as spinach,
dandelion, turnip, mustard, Swiss
chard

½ teaspoon salt

¼ cup water

1 tablespoon minced fresh chervil
or 1 teaspoon dried tarragon

1 tablespoon chopped fresh parsley

3 cups water

1 teaspoon salt

1 teaspoon finely grated lemon rind
(yellow part only)

1 cup fine-ground cornmeal

1 teaspoon olive oil

Freshly ground black pepper

1. In a large pot, heat the olive oil over medium heat. Add the leeks or onions and cook for 5 minutes, or until softened. Stir in the garlic, cook until fragrant, then add the greens and salt. Cook, stirring constantly, until the greens begin to wilt.

2. Add the water and cook, stirring frequently, until the greens are greatly reduced in volume and the water is evaporated, about 10 minutes. Add the chervil or tarragon and parsley. Cook for another minute, and turn off the heat.

3. In a medium-size saucepan, bring the water and salt to a gentle boil. Add the lemon peel and, stirring constantly, add the cornmeal gradually by letting it trickle through your fingers in a slow, steady stream. Stir vigorously, making sure to scrape the bottom of the pan. Break apart any lumps that form. The polenta is done when it is the consistency of thick porridge and begins to pull away from the side of the pan, about 5 to 10 minutes.

4. Mix the polenta with the mixed greens and immediately pour the mixture into a greased 10-inch pie plate. Allow the pie to set for about 10 minutes, until it firms up.

5. Meanwhile, preheat the broiler. Drizzle the olive oil over the pie, season with the pepper, and broil until the top is tightly crusted, about 3 minutes.

Used with permission from Laura Greenspan, *The Genesis Farm Cookbook.*

Squash and Cranberry Bake

2 cups butternut winter squash,
  peeled, seeded, and cubed
Salt and freshly ground pepper
3 tablespoons soft margarine

1 tablespoon white onion, chopped
2 tablespoons brown sugar, packed
¾ cup cranberries, halved
⅛ teaspoon ground nutmeg

1. Place squash in salted boiling water; cover and cook for 10 minutes or until tender. Do not overcook. Drain well.
2. Preheat oven to 400°F. In a large bowl, mash hot squash and beat with salt and pepper, 2 tablespoons of margarine, onion, and brown sugar. Stir in cranberries. Place mixture in a 1- to 1½-quart baking dish, sprinkle with nutmeg, and dot with remaining margarine. Bake for 45 minutes and serve. Leftovers can be frozen.

Used with permission from the Ellsworth Cooking School, Ellsworth, Maine.

Vegetables Roasted with Garlic and Fresh Basil

3 large onions, sliced thin

5 bell peppers, a mixture of red and green, cut into 2½-inch strips

6 medium zucchini and other summer squash, cut into 2½-inch strips

1 large or two small purple eggplants, cut into 2½-inch strips

7 large cloves garlic, finely minced

2 cups fresh basil leaves, coarsely chopped

¼ cup extra-virgin olive oil

1 teaspoon salt

Freshly ground black pepper

6 large tomatoes, peeled and seeded

1. Preheat oven to 450°F.
2. In a large roasting pan, mix all the vegetables except the tomatoes. Add 4 cloves garlic, 1 cup basil, olive oil, salt, and pepper. Coat the vegetables well, put in the oven and roast, uncovered, for about 30 minutes, stirring occasionally. The vegetables should be lightly browned and most of the liquid evaporated.
3. Add the tomatoes and roast for another 30 minutes, stirring occasionally. Stir in the remaining basil and garlic, and roast for another 15 minutes.

These vegetables can be served alone or with a sprinkling of Parmesan cheese, over pasta, tossed with tofu, Italian sausages, or served at room temperature in pitas with a slice of mozzarella cheese.

> **Serves 4.**
> Nutritional analysis, per serving: calories, 350; fat, 16g; cholesterol, 0mg; carbohydrate, 49g; fiber, 17g; protein, 12g; calories from fat, 26%

Used with permission from Laura Greenspan, *The Genesis Farm Cookbook*.

BREAKFAST DISHES

Buckwheat Banana Pancakes with Blueberry Sauce

1 cup buckwheat pancake/waffle
mix

1 cup water
1 large banana, mashed

1. In a medium-size bowl, blend the pancake mix, water, and banana with an electric hand mixer.
2. Meanwhile, preheat a nonstick griddle or skillet to 450°F. Pour the pancake mixture onto the griddle and cook for 1½ to 2½ minutes. Then turn the pancakes over and cook for another minute. Transfer the pancakes to a plate and serve with blueberry sauce (below).

Variation: We suggest French Acadian Buckwheat pancake mix from Bouchards Family Farm, www.ployes.com.

Serves 2.
Nutritional analysis, per serving: calories, 275; fat, 3g; cholesterol, 0mg; fiber, 9g; protein, 13g; calories from fat, 10%

Blueberry Sauce

1 cup fresh or frozen blueberries
2 tablespoons orange juice

1 teaspoon maple syrup

In a microwave-safe bowl, combine the blueberries, orange juice, and maple syrup. Microwave on medium setting for 5 minutes. Drizzle over the pancakes.

Serves 2.
Nutritional analysis, per serving: calories, 56; fat, 0g; cholesterol, 0mg; carbohydrate, 14g; fiber, 2g; protein, 1g; calories from fat, 0%

Courtesy of Daniel Nadeau, M.D.

Free-Range Confetti Omelet

1 tablespoon canola oil

1 medium-size onion, chopped

¼ cup red bell peppers, chopped

¼ cup green bell peppers, chopped

½ cup mushrooms, sliced

1 medium-size tomato, chopped

1 green chili pepper, seeded and chopped

¼ teaspoon salt

⅛ teaspoon freshly ground pepper

4 large free-range eggs

1 tablespoon water

1. In an omelet pan or small skillet, heat the oil over medium-high heat. Add the vegetables, salt, and pepper, and cook, stirring frequently, for 3 to 5 minutes, until the vegetables are very tender. Transfer the vegetables to a plate; cover and set aside.
2. In a small bowl, whisk together the eggs and water. Coat the same skillet with cooking spray and heat over medium-high heat. Pour in the egg mixture all at once.
3. With a metal spatula, gently push the cooked edges of the omelet toward the center of the pan, allowing the uncooked portion of egg to flow underneath, until the egg thickens and no liquid remains.
4. When the underside of the omelet begins to brown, spoon the cooked vegetable mixture onto one half of the omelet. With a spatula, fold the omelet in half or roll one side of the omelet over the filling. Serve immediately.

Serves 4.
Nutritional analysis, per serving: calories, 130; fat, 9g; cholesterol, 215mg; carbohydrate, 6g; fiber, 1g; protein, 7g; calories from fat, 13%

Courtesy of Daniel Nadeau, M.D.

Zucchini, Red Pepper, and Leek Frittata

••

3 small zucchini, thinly sliced
1 red pepper, diced
1 leek, white part only, sliced
2 cups egg substitute, divided

¼ teaspoon black pepper, divided
½ teaspoon dried thyme, divided
Vegetable or olive-oil spray

1. Steam or microwave the vegetables together until tender; they will all cook at the same approximate rate. Set aside.
2. Preheat oven to 350°F. Spray a light coat of oil on a heavy ovenproof skillet. Heat oil over medium heat and add half the egg substitute. Sprinkle it with half the thyme and half the black pepper. Let it cook for a few seconds, until it begins to bubble, and then use a spatula to pull the sides in and spread the uncooked egg over the bottom of the pan, as if cooking an omelet.
3. When this is nearly cooked, add steamed vegetables to pan. Evenly pour in the remaining half of the egg substitute, and sprinkle with the remaining thyme and black pepper. Bake for 35 to 40 minutes, until egg is firm. Serve immediately.

Serves 6.
Nutritional analysis, per serving: calories, 92; fat, 3g; cholesterol, 1mg; fiber, 1g; calories from fat, 27%

Used with permission from the Produce for Better Health Foundation.

DESSERTS

Blueberry Granola Bars

½ cup honey

¼ cup firmly packed brown sugar

3 tablespoons vegetable oil

1½ teaspoons ground cinnamon

1½ cups quick-cooking oats

2 cups fresh blueberries

1. Preheat oven to 350°F. Lightly grease a 9 × 9-inch square baking pan.
2. In a medium-size saucepan, combine honey, brown sugar, oil, and cinnamon, and bring to a boil. Continue boiling for 2 minutes; do not stir.
3. In a large mixing bowl, combine oats and blueberries. Stir in honey mixture until thoroughly blended. Spread into the prepared baking pan, gently pressing mixture flat. Bake until lightly browned, about 40 minutes. Cool completely in the pan on a wire rack. Cut into 1½ by 3-inch bars.

Makes 18 bars.
Nutritional analysis, per serving: calories, 97; fat, 3g; carbohydrate, 17g; protein, 1g; calories from fat, 28%

Used with permission from the North American Blueberry Council.

Blueberry-Pineapple Parfait

. . . .

1 can (20 ounces) pineapple
  chunks, drained
1 container (8 ounces) lemon-
  flavored fat-free yogurt

1½ cups fresh or thawed frozen
  blueberries, patted dry
½ cup granola

In a small bowl, combine the pineapple with half the yogurt. In small wineglasses or juice glasses, alternately layer the pineapple-yogurt mixture, blueberries, and granola. Repeat the layering twice. Top each parfait with a dollop of yogurt.

> **Serves 4.**
> Nutritional analysis, per serving: calories, 233; fat, 3g; cholesterol, 0mg; carbohydrate, 49g; fiber, 3g; protein, 4g; calories from fat, 12%

Used with permission from the North American Blueberry Council.

Blueberry Sorbet

. . . .

4 cups fresh or thawed frozen
  blueberries

1 can (6 ounces) frozen apple juice
  concentrate

1. In a food processor or blender, combine blueberries and apple juice concentrate; blend until liquefied. Pour into an 11- by 17-inch baking pan. Cover and freeze until firm around the edges, about 2 hours.
2. With a heavy spoon, break frozen mixture into pieces. In a food processor or blender container, place mixture and blend until smooth but not completely melted. Spoon into a 9-by 5-inch loaf pan; cover and freeze until firm. Serve within a few days.

> **Serves 6.**
> Nutritional analysis, per serving: calories, 112; fat, 1g; carbohydrate, 28g; protein, 1g; calories from fat, 8%

Used with permission from the North American Blueberry Council.

SMOOTHIES

Dan's Blueberry-Banana Smoothie

· ·

1 cup soy milk

1 cup unsweetened fresh or frozen
blueberries

1 large banana

1 teaspoon dried flaxseed/linseed

In a blender container, combine soy milk, blueberries, banana, and flaxseed/linseed. Blend until smooth.

> **Serves 1.**
>
> Nutritional analysis, per serving: calories, 301; fat, 7g; cholesterol, 0mg; carbohydrate, 56g; fiber, 11g; protein, 10g; calories from fat, 21%

Courtesy of Daniel Nadeau, M.D.

Mango Smoothie

· ·

1 cup fresh or frozen mango, sliced

1 cup unsweetened soy milk

½ large banana

In a blender container, combine mango, soy milk, and banana; blend until smooth.

> **Serves 1.**
>
> Nutritional analysis, per serving: calories, 251; fat, 5g; cholesterol, 0mg; carbohydrate, 48g; fiber, 8g; protein, 9g; calories from fat, 18%

Courtesy of Daniel Nadeau, M.D.

Paradise Freeze

• •

1 large, ripe banana
1 cup strawberries
1 ripe mango, cubed

1 cup cranberry juice
1 cup ice cubes

In a blender or food processor, combine banana, strawberries, mango, cranberry juice, and ice cubes. Cover; blend until thick and smooth.

Serves 3.
Nutritional analysis, per serving: calories, 131; fat, 1g; cholesterol, 0mg; carbohydrate, 41g; protein, 1g; calories from fat, 7%

Used with permission from Dole Food Company, Inc.

BIBLIOGRAPHY

Chapter 2: Red

Agarwal, S., et al. "Tomato lycopene and low-density lipoprotein oxidation: a human dietary intervention study." *Lipids* 33 (October 1998): 981–84.

Arab, L., et al. "Lycopene and the lung." Presented in abstract at the New York Academy of Medicine, April 10, 2001.

Aviram, A., et al. "Human serum paraoxonases (PON1) Q and R selectively decrease lipid peroxides in human coronary and carotid atherosclerotic lesions: PON esterase and peroxidase-like activities." *Circulation* 101 (May 30, 2000): 2510–17.

Aviram, M. "Does paraoxonase play a role in susceptibility to cardiovascular disease?" *Molecular Medicine Today* 5 (September 1999): 381–86.

Aviram, M., et al. "Pomegranate juice consumption reduces oxidative stress, atherogenic modifications to LDL, and platelet aggregation: studies in humans and in atherosclerotic apolipoprotein E-deficient mice." *American Journal of Clinical Nutrition* 71 (May 2000): 1062–76.

Bernstein, P., et al. "Identification and quantitation of carotenoids and their metabolites in the tissues of the human eye." *Experimental Eye Research* 72 (March 2001): 215–23.

Bickford, P. C., et al. "Effects of aging on cerebellar noradrenergic function and motor learning: nutritional interventions." *Mechanisms of Ageing and Development* 111 (November 1999): 141–54.

Blacklock, C. J., et al. "Salicylic acid in the serum of subject not taking aspirin. Comparison of salicylic acid concentrations in the serum of vegetarians, non-vegetarians, and patients taking low-dose aspirin." *Journal of Clinical Pathology* 54 (July 2001): 553–55.

Cao, G., et al. "Serum antioxidant capacity is increased by consumption of strawberries, spinach, red wine or vitamin C in elderly women." *Journal of Nutrition* 128 (December 1998): 2383–90.

Clinton, S. K. "Tomatoes and prostate cancer: integration of basic and clinical studies." Presented in abstract at the New York Academy of Medicine, April 10, 2001.

Eberhardt, M. V., et al. "Antioxidant activity of fresh apples." *Nature* 405 (June 22, 2000): 903–4.

Gann, P., et al. "Lower prostate cancer risk in men with elevated plasma lycopene levels: results of a prospective analysis." *Cancer Research* 59 (March 15, 1999): 1225–30.

Gartner, C., et al. "Lycopene is more bioavailable from tomato paste than from fresh tomatoes." *American Journal of Clinical Nutrition* 66 (July 1997): 116–22.

Giovanucci, E., et al. "Intake of carotenoids and retinol in relation to risk of prostate cancer." *Journal of the National Cancer Institute* 87 (December 6, 1995): 1767–76.

Hertog, M., et al. "Dietary antioxidant flavonoids and risk of coronary heart disease: the Zutphen Elderly Study." *Lancet* 342 (October 23, 1993): 1007–11.

Hertog, M., et al. "Antioxidant flavonols and coronary heart disease risk." (Letter) *Lancet* 349 (1997): 699.

Hesler, M. A., et al. "Influence of fruit and vegetable juices on the endogenous formation of N-nitrosoproline and N-nitrosothiazolidine-4-carboxylic acid in humans on controlled diets." *Carcinogenesis* 13 (December 1992): 2277–80.

Howell, A. B., et al. "Inhibition of the adherence of p-fimbriated *Escherichia coli* to uroepithelial-cell surfaces by proanthocyanidin extracts from cranberries." *New England Journal of Medicine* 339 (October 8, 1998): 1085–86.

Kapadia, G. J., et al. "Chemoprevention of lung and skin cancer by Beta vulgaris (beet) root extract." *Cancer Letters* 100 (1–2) (February 27, 1996): 211–14.

Knekt, P. "Dietary flavonoids and the risk of lung cancer and other malignant neoplasms." *American Journal of Epidemiology*, 146 (August 1, 1997): 223–30.

Knekt, P., et al. "Quercetin intake and the incidence of cerebrovascular disease." *European Journal of Clinical Nutrition* 54 (May 2000): 415–17.

Le Marchand, L., et al. "Intake of Flavonoids and Lung Cancer." *Journal of the National Cancer Institute* 92 (January 19, 2000): 154–60.

Lewis, S., et al. "The relationship of respiratory symptoms and lung function with intakes of apples and tomatoes." Presented at the 97th annual meeting of the American Thoracic Society in San Francisco, May 20, 2001.

Maas, J. L., et al. "Ellagic acid, an anticarcinogen in fruits, especially in strawberries: a review." *Horticultural Science* 26 (1991): 10–14.

Mee, K. A. "Apple fiber and gum arabic lowers total and low-density lipoprotein cholesterol levels in men with mild hypercholesterolemia." *Journal of the American Dietetic Association* 97 (April 1997): 422–24.

Mühlbauer, R. C., et al. "Effect of vegetables on bone metabolism." *Nature* 401 (September 23, 1999): 343–44.

Snowdon, D. A., et al. "Antioxidants and reduced functional capacity in the elderly: findings from the Nun Study." *Journal of Gerontology: Medical Sciences* 51A (January 1996): M10–M16.

Stoner, J. D., et al. "Isothiocyanates and freeze-dried strawberries as inhibitors of esophageal cancer." *Toxicological Sciences* 52, supp. no. 2 (December 1999): 95–100.

Wang, H., et al. "Antioxidant and anti-inflammatory activities of anthocyanins and their aglycon, cyanidin, from tart cherries." *Journal of Natural Products* 62 (February 1999): 294–96.

———. "Antioxidant polyphenols from tart cherries (*Prunus cerasus*)." *Journal of Agricultural and Food Chemistry* 47 (March 1999): 840–44.

Weiss, E. I., et al. "Inhibiting interspecies coaggregation of plaque bacteria with cranberry juice constituent." *Journal of the American Dental Association* 129 (December 1998): 1719–23.

Wilson, T., et al. "Cranberry extract inhibits low density lipoprotein oxidation." *Life Sciences* 62 (1998): PL 381–86.

Xing, N., et al. "Quercetin inhibits the expression and function of the androgen receptor in LNCaP prostate cancer cells." *Carcinogenesis* 22 (March 2001): 409–14.

Chapter Three: Orange-Yellow

Appel, L. J., et al. "A Clinical Trial of the Effects of Dietary Patterns on Blood Pressure." *New England Journal of Medicine* 336 (April 17, 1997): 1117–24.

Bertram, J. S. "Cellular communications via gap junctions." *Science & Medicine* 7 (March–April 2000): 18–27.

Botting, K. J., et al. "Antimutagens in food plants eaten by Polynesians: micronutrients, phytochemicals and protection against bacterial mutagenicity of the heterocyclic amine 2-amino-3-methylimidazo [4, 5-f] quinoline." *Food and Chemical Toxicology* 37 (2–3) (February–March 1999): 95–103.

Burke, Y. D., et al. "Inhibition of pancreatic cancer growth by the dietary isoprenoids farnesol and geraniol." *Lipids* 32 (February 1997): 151–56.

Carbin, B. E., et al. "Treatment of benign prostatic hyperplasia with phytosterols." *British Journal of Urology* 66 (December 1990): 639–41.

Chiang, M-Y, et al. "An essential role for retinoid receptors RARbeta and RXRgamma in long-term potentiation and depression." *Neuron* 21 (December 1998): 1353–61.

Dorgan, J. F., et al. "Relationships of serum carotenoids, retinol, alpha-tocopherol, and selenium with breast cancer risk: results from a prospective study in Columbia, Missouri (United States)." *Cancer Causes and Control* 9 (January 1998): 89–97.

Gaziano, J. M., et al. "A prospective study of consumption of carotenoids in fruits and vegetables and decreased cardiovascular mortality in the elderly." *Annals of Epidemiology* 5 (July 1995) 255–60.

Goodman, M. T., et al. "The association of plasma micronutrients with the risk of cervical dysplasia in Hawaii." *Cancer Epidemiology, Biomarkers and Prevention* 7 (June 1998): 537–44.

Hakim, I. A., et al. "Assessing dietary D-limonene intake for epidemiological studies." *Journal of Food Composition and Analysis* 13 (August 2000): 329–36.

Howard, A. N., et al. "Do hydroxy-carotenoids prevent coronary heart disease? A comparison between Belfast and Toulouse." *International Journal of Vitamin and Nutritional Research* 66 (1996): 113–18.

Inserra, P. F., et al. "Immune function in elderly smokers and nonsmokers improves during supplementation with fruit and vegetable extracts." *Integrative Medicine* 2 (1999): 3–10.

Joshipura, K. J., et al. "Fruit and vegetable intake in relation to risk of ischemic stroke." *Journal of the American Medical Association* 282 (October 6, 1999): 1233–39.

Kane, G. C., et al. "Drug-grapefruit interactions." *Mayo Clinic Proceedings* 75 (September 2000): 933–42.

Karanja, N. M., et al. "Descriptive characteristics of the dietary patterns used in the Dietary Approaches to Stop Hypertension trial." *Journal of the American Dietetic Association* 99 (Supp. no. 8) (August 1999): S19–S27.

Le Marchand, L., et al. "Intake of specific carotenoids and lung cancer risk." *Cancer Epidemiology* 2 (May–June 1993): 183–87.

Le Marchand, L., et al. "Intake of flavonoids and lung cancer." *Journal of the National Cancer Institute* 92 (January 19, 2000): 154–60.

Michaud, D. S., et al. "Intake of specific carotenoids and risk of lung cancer in 2 prospective US cohorts." *American Journal of Clinical Nutrition* 72 (October 2000): 990–97.

Murakoshi, M., et al. "Potent preventive action of alpha-carotene against carcinogenesis: spontaneous liver carcinogenesis and promoting stage of lung and skin carcinogenesis in mice are suppressed more effectively by alpha-carotene than by beta-carotene." *Cancer Research* 52 (December 1, 1992): 6583–87.

Nadeau, D. A. "Intestinal warfare: the role of fructooligosaccharides in health and disease." *Nutrition in Clinical Care* 3 (September–October 2000): 266–73.

Robertson, J., et al. "The effect of raw carrot on serum lipids and colon function." *American Journal of Clinical Nutrition* 32 (September 1979): 1889–92.

Santos, M. S., et al. "Natural killer cell activity in elderly men is enhanced by beta-carotene supplementation." *American Journal of Clinical Nutrition* 64 (November 1996): 772–77.

Speizer, F. E., et al. "Prospective study of smoking, antioxidant intake, and lung cancer in middle-aged women (USA)." *Cancer Causes and Control* 10 (October 1999): 475–82.

Steinmetz, K. A., et al. "Vegetables, fruit, and cancer prevention: a review." *Journal of the American Dietetic Association* 96 (October 1996): 1027–39.

Walaszek, Z., et al. "D-Glucaric acid content of various fruits and vegetables and cholesterol-lowering effects of dietary D-glucarate in the rat." *Nutrition Research* 16 (April 1996): 673–81.

Wang, W., et al. "Cell-cycle arrest at G2/M and growth inhibition by apigenin in human colon carcinoma cell lines." *Molecular Carcinogenesis* 28 (June 2000) 102–10.

Yoshimi, N., et al. "Inhibition of azoxymethane-induced rat colon carcinogenesis by potassium hydrogen D-glucarate." *International Journal of Oncology* 16 (January 2000): 43–48.

Zhang, L-X, et al. "Carotenoids up-regulate *connexin 43* gene expression independent of their provitamin A or antioxidant properties." *Cancer Research* 52 (October 15, 1992): 5707–12.

Chapter Four: Green

Bell, M. C., et al. "Placebo-controlled trial of indole-3-carbinol in the treatment of CIN." *Gynecologic Oncology* 78 (August 2000): 123–29.

Brown, L., et al. "A prospective study of carotenoid intake and risk of cataract extraction in US men." *American Journal of Clinical Nutrition* 70 (October 1999): 517–24.

Chasan-Taber, L., et al. "A prospective study of carotenoid and vitamin A intakes and risk of cataract extraction in US women." *American Journal of Clinical Nutrition* 70 (October 1999): 509–16.

Cohen, J. H., et al. "Fruit and vegetable intakes and prostate cancer risk." *Journal of the National Cancer Institute* 92 (January 5, 2000): 61–68.

Colodny, L. R., et al. "The role of esterin processed alfalfa saponins in reducing cholesterol." *Journal of the American Nutraceutical Association* 3 (Winter 2001): 6–15.

Dagnelie, G., et al. "Lutein improves visual function in some patients with retinal degeneration: a pilot study via the Internet." *Optometry* 71 (March 2000): 147–64.

Duffy, S. J., et al. "Short- and long-term black tea consumption reverses endothelial dysfunction in patients with coronary artery disease." *Circulation* 104 (July 10, 2001): 151–56.

Dulloo, A. G., et al. "Efficacy of a green tea extract rich in catechin polyphenols and caffeine in increasing 24-hour energy expenditure and fat oxidation in humans." *American Journal of Clinical Nutrition* 70 (December 1999): 1040–45.

Dulloo, A. G., et al. "Green tea and thermogenesis: interactions between catechin-polyphenols, caffeine and sympathetic activity." *International Journal of Obesity and Related Metabolic Disorders* 24 (February 2000): 252–58.

Dwyer, J. H., et al. "Oxygenated carotenoid lutein and progression of early athersclerosis: the Los Angeles Atherosclerosis Study." *Circulation* 103 (June 19, 2001): 2922–27.

Edenharder, R., et al. "Isolation and characterization of structurally novel antimutagenic flavonoids from spinach (*Spinacia oleracea*)." *Journal of Agricultural and Food Chemistry* 49 (June 2001): 2767–73.

Englisch, W., et al. "Efficacy of artichoke dry extract in patients with hyperlipoproteinemia." *Arzneimittelforschung* 50 (March 2000): 260–65.

Fahey, J. W., et al. "Broccoli sprouts: an exceptionally rich source of inducers of enzymes that protect against chemical carcinogens." *Pro-*

ceedings of the National Academy of Sciences 94 (September 1997): 10367–72.

Fahey, J. W., et al. "Antioxidant functions of sulforaphane: a potent inducer of phase II detoxication enzymes." *Food and Chemical Toxicology* 37 (9–10) (September–October 1999): 973–79.

Flagg, E. W., et al. "Dietary glutathione intake and the risk of oral and pharyngeal cancer." *American Journal of Epidemiology* 139 (March 1, 1994): 453–65.

Fowke, J. H., et al. "*Brassica* vegetable consumption shifts estrogen metabolism in healthy postmenopausal women." *Cancer Epidemiology, Biomarkers and Prevention* 9 (August 2000): 773–79.

Gamet-Payrastre, L., et al. "Sulforaphane, a naturally occurring isothiocyanate, induces cell cycle arrest and apoptosis in HT29 human colon cancer cells." *Cancer Research* 60 (March 1, 2000): 1426–35.

Geleijnse, J. M., et al. "Tea flavonoids may protect against atherosclerosis: the Rotterdam Study." *Archives of Internal Medicine* 159 (October 11, 1999): 2170–74.

Hakim, I. A., et al. "Tea intake and squamous cell carcinoma of the skin: influence of type of tea beverages." *Cancer Epidemiology, Biomarkers and Prevention* 9 (July 2000): 727–31.

Hammond, B. R., Jr., et al. "Preservation of visual sensitivity of older subjects: association with macular pigment density." *Investigative Ophthalmology and Visual Science* 39 (February 1998): 397–406.

Hecht, S. S., et al. "Effects of watercress consumption on metabolism of a tobacco-specific lung carcinogen in smokers." *Cancer Epidemiology, Biomarkers and Prevention* 4 (December 1995): 877–84.

Hertog, M. G., et al. "Antioxidant flavonols and ischemic heart disease in a Welsh population of men: the Caerphilly Study." *American Journal of Clinical Nutrition* 65 (May 1997): 1489–94.

Huanbiao, M., et al. "Farnesyl anthranilate suppresses the growth, in vitro and in vivo, of murine B16 melanomas." *Cancer Letters* 157 (September 1, 2000): 145–53.

Joshipura, K. J., et al. "Fruit and vegetable intake in relation to risk of ischemic stroke." *Journal of the American Medical Association* 282 (October 6, 1999): 1233–39.

Keli, S. O., et al. "Dietary flavonoids, antioxidant vitamins, and incidence of stroke: the Zutphen study." *Archives of Internal Medicine* 156 (March 25, 1996): 637–42.

Le Marchand, L., et al. "An ecological study of diet and lung cancer in the South Pacific." *International Journal of Cancer* 53 (September 7, 1995): 118–23.

London, S. J., et al. "Isothiocyanates, glutathione S-transferase M1 and T1 polymorphisms, and lung-cancer risk: a prospective study of men in Shanghai, China." *Lancet* 356 (August 26, 2000): 724–29.

Lu, Y-P, et al. "Stimulatory effect of oral administration of green tea or caffeine on ultraviolet light-induced increases in epidermal wild-type p53, p21(WAF1/CIP1), and apoptotic sunburn cells in SKH-1 mice." *Cancer Research* 60 (September 1, 2000): 4785–91.

———. "Inhibitory effect of black tea on the growth of established skin tumors in mice: Effects on tumor size, apoptosis, mitosis, and bromodeoxyuridine incorporation into DNA." *Carcinogenesis* 18 (November 1997): 2163–69.

Sato, Y., et al. "Possible contribution of green tea drinking habits to the prevention of stroke." *Tohoku Journal of Experimental Medicine* 157 (April 1989): 337–43.

Seddon, J. M., et al. "Dietary carotenoids, vitamins A, C, and E, and advanced age-related macular degeneration." *Journal of the American Medical Association* 272 (November 9, 1994): 1413–20.

Taniguchi, S., et al. "Effect of (-)-epigallocatechin gallate, the main constituent of green tea, on lung metastasis with mouse B16 melanoma cell lines." *Cancer Letters* 65 (July 31, 1992): 51–4.

Xu, D., et al. "Homocysteine accelerates endothelial cell senescence." *FEBS Letters (Federation of European Biochemical Societies)* 470 (March 17, 2000): 20–4.

Yochum, L., et al. "Dietary flavonoid intake and risk of cardiovascular disease in postmenopausal women." *American Journal of Epidemiology* 149 (May 15, 1999): 943–49.

Zhang, Y., et al. "Anticarcinogenic activities of sulforaphane and structurally related synthetic norbornyl isothiocyanates." *Proceedings of the National Academy of Sciences* 91 (April 12, 1994): 3147–50.

Chapter Five: Blue-Purple

Bickford, P. C., et al. "Antioxidant-rich diets improve cerebellar physiology and motor learning in aged rats." *Brain Research* 866 (1–2) (June 2, 2000): 211–17.

Bomser, J., et al. "In vitro anticancer activity of fruit extracts form Vaccinium species." *Planta Medica* 62 (June 1996): 212–16.

Freedman, J. E., et al. "Select flavonoids and whole juice from purple grapes inhibit platelet function and enhance nitric oxide release." *Circulation* 103 (June 12, 2001): 2792–98.

Joseph, J. A., et al. "Reversals of age-related declines in neuronal signal transduction, cognitive, and motor behavioral deficits with blueberry, spinach, or strawberry dietary supplementation." *Journal of Neuroscience* 19 (September 15, 1999): 8114–21.

Karandeniz, F., et al. "Polyphenolic composition of raisins." *Journal of Agricultural and Food Chemistry* 48 (November 20, 2000): 5343–50.

Keevil, J. G., et al. "Grape juice, not orange juice or grapefruit juice, inhibits human platelet aggregation." *Journal of Nutrition* 130 (January 2000): 53–6.

Leitner, G., et al. "Stress induced electrolyte and blood gas changes with and without a six day oral treatment with elderberry concentrate." *Magnesium Bulletin* 22 (September 2000): 72–9.

Morazzoni, P., et al. "*Vaccinium myrtillus L.*" *Fitoterapia* 67 (1996): 3–29.

Purba, M., et al. "Skin wrinkling: can food make a difference?" *Journal of the American College of Nutrition* 20 (February 2001): 71–80.

Stein, J. H., et al. "Purple grape juice improves endothelial function and reduces the susceptibility of LDL cholesterol to oxidation in patients with coronary artery disease." *Circulation* 100 (September 7, 1999): 1050–55.

Youdim, K. A., et al. "Incorporation of the elderberry anthocyanins by endothelial cells increases protection against oxidative stress." *Free Radical Biology and Medicine* 29 (July 1, 2000): 51–60.

Zakay-Rones, Z., et al. "Inhibition of several strains of influenza virus *in vitro* and reduction of symptoms by an elderberry extract (*Sambucus nigra L.*) during an outbreak of influenza B Panama." *Journal of Alternative and Complementary Medicine* 1 (Winter 1995): 361–69.

Chapter Six: The Eating Program

Fraser, G. E., et al. "A possible protective effect of nut consumption on risk of coronary heart disease. The Adventist Health Study." *Archives of Internal Medicine* 152 (July 1992): 1416–24.

Haggans, C. J., et al. "Effect of flaxseed consumption on urinary estrogen metabolites in postmenopausal women." *Nutrition and Cancer* 32 (1999): 188–95.

Hu, F. B., et al. "Frequent nut consumption and risk of coronary heart disease in women: prospective cohort study." *British Medical Journal* 317 (November 14, 1998): 1341–45.

Iso, H., et al. "Intake of fish and omega-3 fatty acids and risk of stroke in women." *Journal of the American Medical Association* 285 (January 17, 2001): 304–12.

Jacobs, D. R., Jr. "Is whole grain intake associated with reduced total and cause-specific death rates in older women? The Iowa Women's Health Study." *American Journal of Public Health* 89 (March 1999): 322–29.

Krauss, R. M., et al. "AHA Dietary Guidelines: revision 2000: a statement for healthcare professionals from the nutrition committee of the American Heart Association." *Stroke* 31 (November 2000): 2751–66.

Liu, S., et al. "Whole grain consumption and risk of ischemic stroke in women: a prospective study." *Journal of the American Medical Association* 284 (September 27, 2000): 1534–40.

Meyer, K. A., et al. "Carbohydrates, dietary fiber, and incident type 2 diabetes in older women." *American Journal of Clinical Nutrition* 71 (April 2000): 921–30.

Sellers, T. A., et al. "Dietary folate intake, alcohol, and risk of breast cancer in a prospective study of postmenopausal women." *Epidemiology* 12 (July 2001): 420–28.

Singh, P. N., et al. "Dietary risk factors for colon cancer in a low-risk population." *American Journal of Epidemiology* 148 (October 15, 1998): 761–74.

INDEX

James A. Joseph, PhD, has conducted research focusing on the effects of nutrition on the anti-aging process for 24 years for the U.S. government, first at the National Institutes of Health, where he held positions as Research Pharmacologist and Senior Staff Fellow of the Gerontology Center; and, since 1993, as Lead Scientist and Lab Chief of the Laboratory of Neuroscience of the USDA Human Nutrition Research Center on Aging at Tufts University in Boston. He has also served as an instructor at Johns Hopkins University Medical School and Tufts University. His academic and professional credentials cover the areas of behavioral neuroscience, biopsychology, and biology.

Daniel Nadeau, MD, MS in Nutrition, is the Medical Director of HealthReach Diabetes, Endocrine and Nutrition Center in Hampton, New Hampshire. Previously, he served as Medical Director of Nutritionals for Abbott International, where he designed new products and implemented multinational clinical trials for the company. His academic interests include nutrition, diabetes, cardiovascular disease, hypertension, and weight management. Concurrent with his medical career, he served for several years as the medical correspondent for WABI-TV, the CBS affiliate in Bangor, Maine.

Anne Underwood is a reporter for *Newsweek*, specializing in health and medicine, and has been with the magazine for 19 years. Her articles have covered the full spectrum of health and medical issues, including asthma, Alzheimer's, alternative medicine, heart disease, bionic body parts, the physical effects of space travel, and the connection between diet and cancer prevention. The first patient to receive the AbioCor artificial heart learned about the device through one of Anne's articles. She graduated from Yale and holds a master's degree from Columbia. Articles she reported have twice been nominated for the prestigious National Magazine Award.